# Head and Neck Nursing

*To Sarah, Matthew, Ellen, Kahra and Kelvin*

*For Churchill Livingstone:*

*Commissioning Editor:* Ninette Premdas
*Project Manager:* Gail Murray
*Project Development Manager:* Dinah Thom

# Head and Neck Nursing

**Michael J. Hahn** BA BDS MDentSc
Oral and Facial Surgery Department, Sunderland Royal Hospital, Sunderland, UK

**Anne Jones** RGN BPSN BSc(Hons)
Oral and Facial Surgery Department, Sunderland Royal Hospital, Sunderland, UK

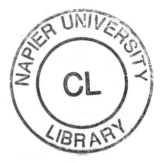

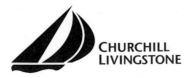

CHURCHILL
LIVINGSTONE

EDINBURGH  LONDON  NEW YORK  PHILADELPHIA  ST LOUIS  SYDNEY  TORONTO  2000

CHURCHILL LIVINGSTONE
An imprint of Harcourt Publishers Limited

© Harcourt Publishers Limited 2000

◢ is a registered trademark of Harcourt Publishers
Limited

The right of Michael J. Hahn and Anne Jones to be identified
as the authors of this work has been asserted by them in
accordance with the Copyright, Designs and Patents Act 1988

First published 2000

ISBN 0 4430 5854 7

**British Library Cataloguing in Publication Data**
A catalogue record for this book is available from the British
Library

**Library of Congress Cataloging in Publication Data**
A catalog record for this book is available from the Library of
Congress

**Note**
Medical knowledge is constantly changing. As new
information becomes available, changes in treatment,
procedures, equipment and the use of drugs become
necessary. The authors and the publishers have, as far as it is
possible, taken care to ensure that the information given in
this text is accurate and up to date. However, readers are
strongly advised to confirm that the information, especially
with regard to drug usage, complies with the latest
legislation and standards of practice.

The
publisher's
policy is to use
**paper manufactured
from sustainable forests**

Printed in China

# Contents

*The plate section is between pages 39 and 40.*

# Preface

In chronological terms the field of head and neck nursing is relatively new, and when we embarked upon writing this book there were no other texts available which were devoted to the subject. Individual subjects were covered, to varying extents, in general nursing works and in books devoted to ENT, dental and plastic surgical nursing. Some of the reasons for this will become apparent in the first chapter of this book, which seeks to describe the development of head and neck surgery from the earliest recorded times to the present day. With the recently developing extended role of nurses, as well as the need for nurses to keep up with the ever-increasing sub-specialisation that is occurring in medical care, we felt that the time for publication of this book was ripe. It was at this point that our difficulties began!

At whom should we aim the book? Initially we thought it would be helpful to have a text of almost pocket size that could be kept in clinical areas that were connected in any way with the head and neck specialty. We hoped it would be read by staff of a wide range of backgrounds and levels of seniority and thus promote one of the concepts that we refer to throughout the book – that of a multidisciplinary approach to patient care. As we proceeded, however, it became very difficult to draw the boundaries. On the one hand we did not want to make the text so general that it would be of no use to postgraduate students on specialist courses, but on the other, we were keen to help colleagues in other areas who may look after head and neck patients only from time to time. We sincerely hope that our solution reflected in the book meets the reader's needs.

A second difficulty was in resisting the temptation to stray into the territory of our surgical colleagues, or the other specialties. Clearly, a basic understanding of the medical and surgical techniques to which our patients are subjected is mandatory, but the depth of knowledge required is more difficult to gauge. There are excellent textbooks which cover related areas such as surgery, radiotherapy, speech therapy, dietetics, maxillofacial prosthetics and so on, which can be consulted. We hope, however, that in the subsequent chapters we give enough relevant information for nurses to understand the contribution of other clinicians, thus enabling them to communicate effectively. How, then, do we present this knowledge?

Each chapter is structured in the same way. The *key points* are listed first followed by six sections. There is a short *introduction* to each chapter which usually highlights the reasons why the subject is of particular interest to the head and neck nurse. This is followed by a section on *anatomy and physiology* which should give a firm basis on which to build clinical knowledge. The remaining sections follow the nursing process, i.e., *assessment, planning, implementation and evaluation*, which gives us a system to present information in a way that will be useful for examination purposes. As with any other system there are some disadvantages in this structure. Clinical practice, and patients, do not fit into neat categories and there will be inevitable discrepancies. Furthermore, if the system is followed too rigorously there will be repetition. It is easy to see, for example, that there is not a world of difference between assessment and evaluation. In practice, however, this merely represents the process of clinical audit and we should be trying to 'close the loop'. Notwithstanding these drawbacks we feel that on balance this approach is as good as any as long as it is used critically.

Even within this framework of presentation there are difficulties. What may be obvious to the experienced head and neck nurse in terms of nomenclature and equipment may be new to others. Moreover, the details of protocols and procedures vary from centre to centre. For these reasons we have tried to keep practical details to a minimum and avoid reference to particular commercial products. This information, after all, can be readily gleaned on placements in the clinical setting with little to be gained by didactically recording it.

Where to start other than the beginning? The first chapter puts the current state of the specialty of head and neck nursing in the context of its historical development. Not only is this intended to be of general educational value but it illustrates the recent emergence of the discipline as a well-defined area of nursing. Subsequent chapters deal with nursing problems that are pre-eminent in the head and neck field. The first of these chapters needs no justification: the importance of airway management is obvious in any clinical setting but in no other field do the pathology and the treatment conspire to present such a challenge to the nurse. Similarly with the chapters on communication problems, psychosocial problems and mouth care – the significance of them is clear to the specialist nurse. What of the other subjects that are covered? There are many commendable books on pain control, wound care and nutritional management. In these subjects we have sought to highlight the areas of specific interest to the head and neck nurse. In so doing we hope to encourage the specialist nurse to ensure that the adapted care administered is based on sound general nursing principles and appropriately researched.

Finally, we would like to remind our readers of two things. Firstly, the information is not comprehensive – to some extent it is personal in that the subjects dealt with are those that occur after some years of working with patients suffering from some of the most devastating illnesses known. Secondly, the information is not static and will date with time. Our hope is that our readers will discuss it, develop it, add to it and, most of all, use it to enhance their care of head and neck patients.

Michael J. Hahn
Anne Jones

Sunderland 1999

# Acknowledgements

Many people have given generously of their time and resources in the production of this book. It is not possible to name them all individually but that does not diminish our gratitude to them. In particular, we would like to thank staff at Sunderland Royal Hospital, Dudley NHS Trust and City Hospital, Birmingham.

Initial encouragement and support were given by Professor P. Ward-Booth, Professor J. W. Frame and Professor J. S. Goldberg. Others who contributed significantly to the preparation of the manuscript were Ms K. Dobie, Dr A. M. Hahn, Ms F. A. Hall, Ms S. Hardy and Mr R. Jones. Permission to reproduce clinical illustrations was given by Mr I. C. Martin, Mr B. G. Millar, Mr J. M. Ryan and Mr L. F. A. Stassen.

**1**

# The development of the head and neck specialty

'One cannot practise a science well unless one knows its history'
Auguste Comte

---

### KEY POINTS

- Dental decay or worms?
- From tree bark splints to transosseous plates
- From bamboo dental splints to osseointegration
- Head and neck surgery developed from both medical and dental origins
- Head and neck surgical nursing is a recent but well-defined specialty

---

Many people involved in the care of patients with head and neck problems today, especially those who have trained in more recent years, may be tempted to see the specialty of head and neck surgical nursing as a new development. In some ways, of course it is, for it is only within the last decade that the surgical field has become better defined and the nursing profession, recognising this, has established appropriate postgraduate training and education. In other respects, however, the nursing care of these patients is very well established and specialisation has been going on for many years, albeit under the separate categories of ENT nursing, plastic surgical nursing and maxillofacial nursing. Furthermore, as we mentioned in the preface, the basic principles of general nursing most certainly apply to head and neck patients, so one cannot be too didactic in defining the specialist area.

From an historical point of view, however, the development of head and neck nursing has, in common with many other specialties, followed the course of our surgical colleagues. For the sake of general interest and to place this development into context we will briefly outline the history of surgery and, where appropriate, illustrate points of specific head and neck interest. It will become apparent that our fate has been closely linked with the dental as well as the medical profession, so highlights from both backgrounds will also be included. Unfortunately, until the formalisation of nursing care in the post-Nightingale era, much of nursing was carried out by untrained and often uneducated women, making it difficult to incorporate its history into the same picture. We will begin by briefly looking at the earliest known societies, but for a more detailed account we would refer the reader to the authoritative work of Albert Lyons (Lyons & Petrucelli 1978).

In primitive societies surgery consisted mainly of treatment for wounds and injuries to the bones. It is likely that infections would be common, and there is evidence that measures were taken to keep wounds protected and dry. Some Amerindian tribes, for example, placed a strip of tree bark between wound edges, which probably permitted drainage and promoted healing by secondary intention. The treatment of fractures was also relatively sophisticated. Splints were fashioned from wood and hardened hides, with suitable openings to permit treatment of compound fractures. Haemorrhage was controlled by pressure, tourniquet, cautery and styptic plant substances, for ligature of blood vessels was apparently unknown. During surgery drugs were used to reduce the pain, and in Central Africa it is known that a beverage, which may have been alcoholic, was used to lessen consciousness.

## Ancient Egypt

There are four remaining medical papyruses which give us some information about surgery in ancient Egypt. The surgical use of the knife, except for circumcision, is barely discussed, but there were several kinds of blade, including those made from stone, metal or papyrus reed. The opening cuts of embalmers were stitched in at least a few cases, but it is not known if suturing was in widespread use. Interestingly, other studies of mummies also show evidence of severe infections, caries and loose teeth that were wired together and of various dental prostheses. The treatment of most infections of the teeth consisted of applying medications aimed at 'drawing out the worms'. This idea of worms as a cause of tooth disease was also prominent in Mesopotamia and the Far East and continued in Western medicine throughout the Middle Ages and even into recent centuries.

Cauterisation was used for the removal of surface tumours and cysts. The fire drill – a heated sharp utensil – is mentioned as a surgical tool, and there is evidence that other instruments were available. The Egyptians also used an adhesive tape, made by impregnating gums into linen strips, to pull gaping wounds together.

## Ancient China

Although surgery was not one of the five methods of treatment listed in the *Nei Ching* (a great medical compendium written by Yu Hsing, the Yellow Emperor c. 2600 BC) the knife was known and used. Hua T'o, one of the few names mentioned in connection with surgery, treated an arm wound of a famous general by cutting the flesh and scraping the bone. (Apparently the patient played chess during the surgery, demonstrating the correct attitude towards pain!) It is thought that some kind of anaesthesia was often used, wine and drugs like hyoscymus being the commonest. Like the Egyptians, the Ancient Chinese also believed that worms were responsible for dental problems. The *Nei Ching* classified nine types of toothache, which were mainly treated by applying or ingesting drugs. Loose teeth were splinted with bamboo.

## Ancient Greece

Throughout early Greek history the gods and warriors were together engaged in treating the sick, and the healing gods became enshrined in special temples, of which the most famous were those dedicated to Asclepios. These temples originated about the 6th century BC and by the 4th century BC had spread over the mainland and by 295 BC had even reached Rome. Among the warrior-lords mentioned in the *Iliad* and the *Odyssey* were Machaon and Podalirios, the sons of Asclepios. Both treated wounds, but Machaon's name was continued through subsequent centuries as the father of surgery. For the most part, surgery was restricted to external injuries and wounds. On the battlefield, weapons that pierced the body were removed and haemorrhage stopped by bandaging. The wounds were washed and picked clean of debris.

The nature of surgery between the Homeric period and the emergence of the philosopher-scientists in the 6th century BC is not known, but by the times of Hippocrates in the mid-5th century BC a multiplicity of practising healers had come upon the scene. There was no system of licensure or certification before 300 BC, and anyone except a woman could take the title of physician. What we consider today branches of medicine were all combined as one healing art. We know that manipulations to reduce dislocations and fractures achieved a high degree of sophistication, sometimes with the employment of mechanical devices. Effective and complex techniques of bandaging all parts of the body are to be found in the works of Hippocrates and in the numerous later commentaries. Cautery was effectively used by the Greeks to treat infections, wounds and tumours. In addition, their careful and extensive use of the knife for operative surgery was impressive.

## Roman times

Greek medicine after Hippocrates reached a peak in Alexandria and shortly afterwards began to infiltrate Rome. Although Roman medicine had a long history of its own, various medical sects from Alexandria were taken to Rome by Greek practitioners and underwent their principal development there. Much of the information of Roman medicine is based on the work of two writers: Cornelius Celsus and Caius Pliny, the Elder, both of the 1st century AD. Celsus was not a medical practitioner but gave outstanding descriptions of surgical procedures. Although best remembered for his description of the characteristics of inflammation – 'rubor et tumor cum calor et dolor' – he also recorded the ligation and division of bleeding vessels. Furthermore, he is credited with the first description of an operation for cancer of the lower lip.

Of all the practitioners, writers and teachers of Roman times the Greek physician Galen (c. 129–200) towered above all. Although much of his work was investigative, clinical and pharmacological, he had an interest in surgical practice. He made suggestions on the use of many instruments, including knives, scissors, forceps, splints and retractors. He also advised on placing incisions and closing them and on draining abscesses.

## Medieval times

During the so-called Dark Ages many of the technical advances of Greco-Roman surgery had been entirely lost because of increasing ignorance of them through disuse. The Muslim schools abandoned many procedures, except the setting of fractures and their favoured use of cautery. Similarly the Christian belief in the mediation of the Holy Ghost as the only possibility for cure led to the gradual abandonment of all but the simplest surgical procedures, such as blood-letting, amputations and dental extractions. Nevertheless, Abulcasis (1013–1107) and Avicenna (908–1036) both described the excision of tumours of the lip with the wound left open to heal by secondary intention.

The re-emergence of surgery in Europe was probably initiated in Italy. Guglielino Salicetti (c. 1210–1277) who was a professor at Bologna and city physician at Verona wrote the first known treatise on regional surgical anatomy. His pupil, Guido Lanfranchi of Milan journeyed to Lyons and Paris, where he did much to establish surgical practice in France.

In the Middle Ages surgery was generally limited to wounds, fractures, dislocations, amputations and the opening of abscesses and fistulas. Many of these procedures, along with blood-letting, tooth-pulling and hair cutting, were carried out by barbers! The Arab tradition of using cautery in preference to ligation persisted. Suturing, often with human hair or thread, was known but rare.

During the Renaissance the development of surgery owed much to France, largely due to Ambroise Paré (1517–1590). This uneducated man was first apprenticed to a barber and later as a wound dresser at the Hôtel-Dieu in Paris. In 1537 he joined the army. Whilst in service he discovered by accident that gunshot wounds healed better with cleansing and dressing than by traditional treatment with boiling oil. During later campaigns Paré achieved haemostasis with ligatures and abandoned cauterising irons. In 1561 he published his treatise *A Universal Surgery* in which many new surgical procedures and apparatus were presented.

## The 17th century

The 17th century, the so-called 'Age of Scientific Revolution', was a major turning point in the history of science, not least in anatomy and physiology. Unfortunately, surgery did not keep pace, and the age of anaesthesia and control of infection had not yet arrived. During this period there were two kinds of surgeon and various grades within the subdivisions. 'True' surgeons concerned themselves with the major operations: suture of holes in the intestines, removal of tumours, plastic operations on the lips and nose and the repair of rectal fistulas. The barber surgeons were wound doctors who also performed blood-letting, the extraction of teeth and the management of fractures, dislocations and external ulcers. In addition there were untutored, itinerant wound doctors who operated for cataracts, bladder stones and hernias – apparently with results so bad that reputable surgeons avoided association with them.

Notwithstanding the general picture described above, there were scattered reports in the 17th century of attempts to excise cancer of the tongue by cautery, or by chain or wire. The first recorded attempt at removal of a cancer of the tongue by cautery was by Marchette in 1664, followed by Wiseman in 1676. Others attempted to cause a cancerous portion of the tongue to slough off by strangulation with heavy ligatures.

## The emergence of dentistry as a profession

As well as the legitimate barber surgeons mentioned above, apothecaries, quacks and indeed anyone who had the skills would take care of teeth. Tooth drawers often displayed their techniques in the street before audiences of passers by (Fig. 1.1). In 1699 an edict of Louis XIV established the professional status of dentists in France. Two years of study were required, followed by an examination before the College of Surgeons on theory and practice. In addition, a special category was created for surgeons who specialised in dentistry.

Dentistry really began its independence with the work of Pierre Fauchard (1678–1761). He collated the considerable body of information

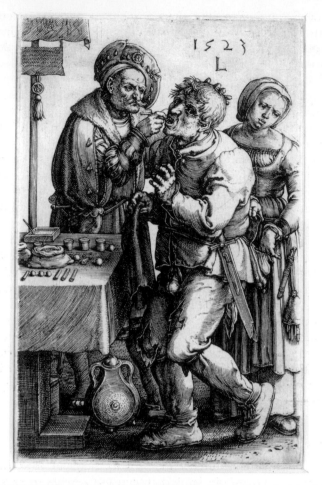

**Figure 1.1**   Dentist treating a patient in *The Toothpuller* by Lucas van Lyden, dated 1523. Reproduced with permission from the Rijksmuseum, Amsterdam.

that had accumulated through the centuries and described the use of tin and lead for filling cavities, but more importantly he established the ethical principle that secret methods should be reported in detail so that the results could be evaluated and used by others. Fauchard's *The Surgeon Dentist* (1728), which became the authoritative text for generations, was the foundation of subsequent dentistry. Nevertheless, dentistry still remained a form of public entertainment. Writings by others in France followed rapidly. Mouton constructed the first gold crowns and Duchâteau, an apothecary in the region of Sèvres, moulded the first porcelain dentures.

   In Germany, incidental dissertations on the teeth by physicians and surgeons were replaced by reports from specialists such as the dentist to

Frederick the Great, Phillip Pfaff, who in 1755 described how to make plaster models from impressions in wax. The craftsmen (usually woodworkers) who actually fashioned the prostheses were the forerunners of dental technicians.

## The 18th century

William Cheseldon (1688–1752) and Percival Pott (1714–1788) dominated surgery during this century. Apart from being gifted surgeons themselves they trained John Hunter (1728–1793), who has been called the founder of experimental surgery and pathology. Possibly his greatest contribution to operative surgery was a new method of closing aneurysms, thus preserving the limbs of thousands by preventing unnecessary amputations.

Among the prominent continental surgeons of this century were Jean-Louis Petit (1674–1760), the inventor of the screw tourniquet, and Pierre Desault (1744–1795), whose bandage for fractured clavicle is still in use today. In Italy Antonio Scarpa (1752–1832) devised a successful operation for inguinal hernia. The German Lorenz Heister (1683–1758) wrote one of the first systemic illustrated textbooks on surgery (1713).

As a result of the work of these men, and of course many others, the surgeons of England and France finally managed to achieve a position of equality with their traditional rivals, the physicians. In 1745, the corporation of surgeons was formally separated from the barbers, but it was not until the last year of the century that the Royal College of Surgeons was finally granted a charter.

## The 19th and 20th centuries

With the development of effective anaesthesia, surgical procedures multiplied in number and complexity. The potential benefits of surgery, however, were overshadowed by the frequent, devastating infections which followed. Only when the principles of asepsis had been established, notably by Lister, were there further developments in surgery. In the late 19th century, perhaps the outstanding surgical innovator in Europe was Albert Christian Theodor Billroth (1829–1894). A German, educated in Berlin, he made his principal contributions in Zurich and then in Vienna, where he was the first to successfully perform extensive operations on the pharynx, larynx and stomach. Unfortunately, his first total laryngectomy patient (1873) died of recurrent disease 8 months later and, in fact, of his first 25 surgical patients before 1890, not one survived a year. On the other hand, Solis Cohen performed the first American laryngectomy in Philadelphia in 1884 and the patient survived for 11 years. Another patient on whom he performed a laryngectomy in 1894 was the first patient on whom oesophageal speech was reported.

Laryngectomy gained favour during the first part of the 20th century due to the efforts of St Clair Thomson in the United Kingdom and Chevalier Jackson in the United States. By 1926 MacKenty was able to report on 100 cases with an operative mortality of only 4%. By 1947 preservation of the voice was being considered and Alonzo of Uruguay described the supraglottic laryngectomy. While this procedure could preserve the voice in carefully selected patients without jeopardising the cure rate, a major contribution was made by Mark Singer and Eric Blom in 1989. They devised the technique of tracheo-oesophageal puncture and the introduction of a valve that allowed total laryngectomy patients to have a reasonable form of speech using pulmonary driven air. Another means of preserving the voice is the early treatment of glottic lesions with $CO_2$ laser using microlaryngoscopy, which is in widespread use today.

Other head and neck procedures were developed around this time, notably the sectioning of the mandible to provide intraoral exposure by Sedillot in 1866, who split the lip and the mandible in the midline. Kocher (1880) described a submandibular approach, and Liston in *Practical Surgery* briefly mentions operations for tumours of the lip, tongue, jaws, thyroid and parotid. The latter surgeon, however, stated that 'the patient with cancer of the antrum may be numbered among the dead' and that surgical treatment 'is totally inadmissible; it is a piece of unmeaning and entirely useless cruelty'. Indeed as late as 1908, Mosher referred to operations for cancer of the paranasal sinuses as 'palliative' only.

One of the great turning points of head and neck surgery was the publication of Crile's work on neck dissection in 1906. Progress was delayed at this time because the operations were lacking in safety and treatment with radiation was thought to be more effective. Nevertheless, the complications of aggressive radiotherapy were significant, and Grant Ward and Hayes Martin arose as strong advocates of radical surgery. Typically, a major head and neck resection would involve hemimandibulectomy, radical neck dissection, resection of the primary tumour and tracheostomy. This description was modified in 1942 to the 'Commando' procedure with a suffix to denote the primary site, e.g. 'Commando – base of tongue' (after the Allied raids on Dieppe the Commandos were recognised as courageous heroes). Grant Ward later modified this to 'composite resection', as the former term suggested an undignified assault on the patient!

The first major step away from the radical neck dissection was the limited neck dissection advocated by the Argentinian Suarez for patients without evidence of clinical neck node metastasis. Eventually there was acceptance that these selective techniques were associated with less morbidity than radical dissections. Clearer classification systems for head and neck malignancy along with remarkable advances in imaging techniques such as computerised tomography (CT) and magnetic resonance (MR) scanning have further improved the management of the disease.

Recognition of the bad prognostic significance of extracapsular spread and the value of adjuvant radiotherapy has also greatly enhanced survival rates in these patients.

There are numerous others who have contributed to the development of head and neck surgery. Lewis described the first complete resection of the temporal bone for carcinoma in 1981, and his operation remains standard practice for treatment of this tumour. Mohs' work has allowed the resection of both small and large cutaneous tumours while having the opportunity to preserve form and function in these patients.

As surgical techniques became more radical, the need for appropriate reconstructive measures was highlighted. In 1964 Bakamjian of Buffalo, USA described the non-delayed deltopectoral flap based medially on perforators in the internal mammary artery. This flap heralded the era of immediate reconstruction in head and neck surgery but it was largely superseded by the introduction of the pectoralis major myocutaneous flap by Ariyan of Yale in 1979. In more recent years, arterialised free tissue transfer from various areas in the body have gained widespread use in reconstruction of the head and neck. Flaps containing bone such as the radial forearm flap, the fibular flap and the iliac crest flap are used for intra-oral reconstruction, particularly when the mandible has been removed.

Apart from these tremendous advances in head and neck surgery *per se* there is no doubt that the two world wars had an enormous influence upon the rate of these developments. Jaques Joseph (1865–1934) on the German side and Sir Harold Gillies in the UK both treated hundreds of disfigured war casualties and invented, sometimes on the spot, many of the procedures that make up the repertoire of head and neck surgeons today. Although these two men were the leading lights at the time, surgeons of many specialties – otolaryngologists, oral surgeons, general surgeons, ophthalmologists and neurosurgeons – worked together to deal with the horrendous deformities that resulted from modern warfare. Unfortunately, after the wars this unity was lost and the plastic surgeons, otolaryngologists and the oral surgeons parted company and often acrimoniously competed for surgical territory, no doubt to the detriment of progress and ultimately patient care.

## The development of dentistry and orthognathic surgery

From the 17th century onwards dentistry gradually became a separate specialty in most countries but it was in the USA that it realised its fullest development. Horace H. Haydon (1768–1864) and Chapin C. Harris (1809–1860) were the main instigators of this progress but there is no doubt that the introduction of general anaesthesia for dental use was a major factor.

The first dental school in the world was established in 1839 as the Baltimore College of Dental Surgery. Interestingly, by 1870, although there were ten thousand dentists in the USA, only one thousand were graduates of a school.

Advances in prostheses, such as the production of vulcanite by Charles Goodyear in 1855 (Fig. 1.2), technical innovations in the management of cavities, improvements in the correction of occlusal discrepancies, and the elevation of educational standards gave American dentistry world leadership. In most countries, however, the specialisation of dentistry, with its complex techniques, became so complete that it was separated from medical practice altogether.

One area of head and neck surgery that retained the interest of both the medical and dental specialties was that of orthognathic surgery. The first operation for the correction of dental malocclusion was carried out by Hullihen in 1849. Hullihen was a general surgeon who also had a dental training. The cradle of early orthognathic surgery, however, was in St Louis, where the orthodontist Edward Angle (1898) and the surgeon Vilray Blair (1906) worked together. Both were involved in the first described osteotomy of the horizontal ramus for the correction of mandibular prognathism. The two world wars saw pauses in the development of orthognathic surgery as the few maxillofacial surgeons involved were committed to treating facial injuries.

The cradle of modern orthognathic surgery was in central Europe. The founder of the 'Vienna School' was Pichler, succeeded by his pupil Trauner who later moved to Graz. Trauner was the inaugurator of several orthognathic procedures but his main contribution was that he trained Heinz Köle

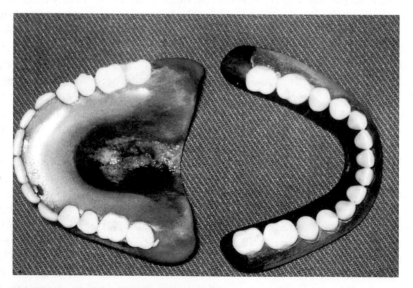

**Figure 1.2**   A set of vulcanite dentures still in use in 1998.

and Hugo Obwegeser who were to become pioneers in orthognathic surgery. In Berlin, Martin Wassmund, who started the 'German School', developed the anterior maxillary osteotomy which is still used today.

American surgeons moved slowly in the direction of orthognathic surgery in the 1950s. Caldwell, Letterman, Robinson, Hinds and Thoma all came up with different methods for the correction of mandibular deformities but it took some time before the Le Fort I and other maxillary and midfacial osteotomies were popularised. It was not until the late 1970s that the USA caught up the Europeans in this area of surgery.

Another step forward in orthognathic surgery was the emergence of bimaxillary surgery – the simultaneous mobilisation of the total maxilla and mandible. Köle had introduced this concept in 1959, and Obwegeser published his experience in 1970 as the first to perform the surgery. It is now routine surgery in many countries, and corrective facial surgery continues to develop, particularly in the craniofacial specialty (Plate 1).

Craniofacial surgery was initially promoted in Europe by Paul Tessier. Although the first Le Fort III osteotomy was performed by Gillies and Harrison in 1942 and another case reported by Gillies and Rowe in 1954, these were isolated cases. Tessier demonstrated spectacular results of his work on severe orbito-craniofacial deformities at a meeting in Rome in 1967.

Much of the progress which has taken place in orthognathic surgery (and, of course, maxillofacial trauma management) has been due to improved methods of fracture fixation. An important catalyst for these changes was the introduction and subsequent widespread use of antibiotic therapy. Before this time closed reduction and indirect skeletal fixation of fractures was the usual treatment of choice. The basic principle of this method of treatment is that the opposing jaw is used as a splint to hold the fractured jaw rigidly in its correct position with the teeth in normal occlusion until bony healing takes place. The fixation is achieved by any one of a number of techniques which generally rely on metal wires or splints attached to the upper and lower dental arches which are in turn secured together to achieve intermaxillary fixation (IMF) (Fig. 1.3).

When satisfactory alignment of the bony fragments could not be achieved with closed reduction, external fixation appliances served to maintain bony fragments in position, frequently without the need for intermaxillary fixation. The commonest external appliances used during that time were pins inserted transcutaneously into the mandible and connected externally by a variety of devices.

Following the introduction of antibiotics, the open treatment of fractures was used more frequently and the controversy arose as to whether or not to use internal fixation devices. Interosseous wire fixation was first used by Buck in the USA in 1847 just after the introduction of ether anaesthesia. The technique was not popularised, however, until the 1940s when a landmark article was published revealing generalised dissatisfaction of surgeons at that

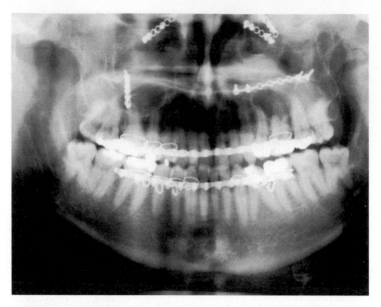

**Figure 1.3**   Panoral radiograph showing arch bars used to achieve intermaxillary fixation. The bars are secured together with elastics or wires with the upper and lower teeth in the correct occlusion for the patient. Until the early 1970s most jaw fractures were reduced and stabilised in this way. The method is still commonly used in some Third World countries.

time with non-operative management of midfacial fractures (Adams 1942).

Attempts to avoid IMF by using more rigid internal fixation devices produced several interesting developments, including metallic mesh implants and bone clamps. The technique most extensively developed, however, and the one most commonly used today is that of fixation with metallic plates and screws (Fig. 1.4).

Bone plates may have been originally introduced into maxillofacial surgery by Christiansen in 1945 when he used tantalum plates to provide interfragmentary stability to unstable mandibular fractures. Further cases of plate and screw fixation were reported sporadically following the Second World War, although until the 1970s most surgeons used plates and screws designed for orthopaedics and applied them to the mandible. Many failures resulted from these early attempts at plate and screw fixation, probably owing to lack of knowledge of the biomechanics of the systems when combined with jaw function. As a result most surgeons limited the use of plates and screws to particular patients, such as epileptics, where postoperative IMF could compromise the airway. Indeed many still used IMF as a supplement.

In the late 1960s and early 1970s several investigators began to adapt much of what had been learned about long bone fractures to those of the mandible. This development was spearheaded by Luhr who designed a

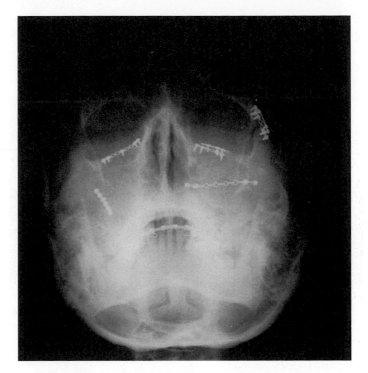

**Figure 1.4**   Open reduction and internal fixation of facial fractures with titanium plates and screws.

vitallium compression plate which was used successfully with IMF. The principles of compression were further utilised by Spiessl whilst he was designing instruments for use in mandibular fracture management. Another simple form of internal fixation, the lag screw, was introduced by Brons and Boering in 1970. In the early 1970s Luhr, Spiessl and most other surgeons used an extraoral approach to fracture fixation although it was recognised that an intraoral approach would eliminate the risk of unsightly facial scars. Intraoral fixation became possible with the miniaturisation of the components. Miniplates and, more recently, microplates are now in widespread use and much current interest centres on the choice of materials. Currently, titanium is the most commonly used material but there is much interest in the search for suitable biodegradable materials to replace it.

Finally, we need to mention the developments that have taken place in maxillofacial reconstruction and prosthetics. As we mentioned earlier, there have been numerous ingenious devices to replace missing teeth from the earliest times, and the use of false noses has been described. As modern surgery has made more radical resection of disease possible and free tissue transfer has greatly enhanced our ability to reconstruct defects, so the development of materials and prosthetic techniques has kept pace. Perhaps the most exciting example of this has been the introduction of osseo-integrated implants. These plasma-coated titanium supports can be placed in bone to support and securely retain prostheses either intraorally (Fig. 1.5) or extraorally (Fig. 1.6). These have been of great benefit not only in terms

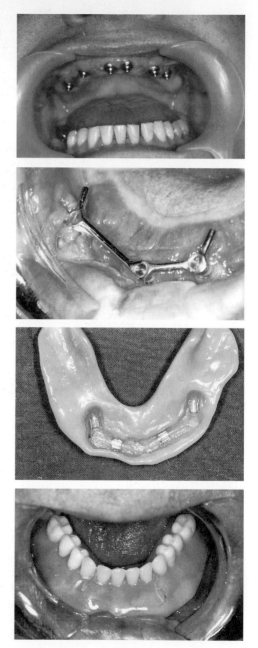

**Figure 1.5** Intraoral implants can be used to support and give retention to dental prostheses. These are particularly helpful to patients who have undergone major resections involving the mouth.

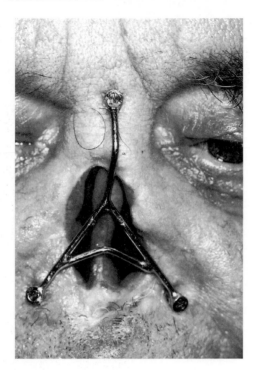

**Figure 1.6**   Extraoral implants are used to retain prostheses which hitherto may have been retained with adhesives or attached to spectacle frames.

of function and aesthetics, but also in the psychological support of patients who previously worried about the embarrassment of their false noses or ears falling off in public, or indeed their dentures displacing during speech.

Clearly no account of such a long period of development of our specialty will be fully comprehensive, but we hope to have applied the 'broad brush strokes' and possibly stimulated an interest for our readers to pursue their own reading. Our main interests, however, lie with the present and future and we will turn our attention to what we perceive as the main areas of significance in the subsequent chapters.

REFERENCES

Adams W M 1942 Internal wiring fixation of social fractures. Surgery 12
Lyons A S, Petrucelli R J 1978 Medicine: an illustrated history. Harry N Abrams, New York

# 2

# Airway management

'No life that breathes with human breath,
Has ever truly longed for death'

Lord Tennyson

---

KEY POINTS

- Emergency airway management
- Tracheostomy
- Epistaxis
- Nasal obstruction

---

## INTRODUCTION

The very basic ethics of our profession require us to be competent in first aid, and by definition this means being able to establish and maintain an airway in the emergency situation. It is tragic that even in recent years there have been well-documented accounts of deaths occurring because patients with bilaterally fractured mandible have been left supine and unattended in the accident and emergency department. Likewise, many hospital staff seem to have an appalling ignorance of even the most basic airway supports.

There is no doubt that even among specialist nurses there is sometimes a lack of confidence in dealing with the airway. To some extent this is understandable – the consequences of mismanagement can be fatal – and there is every reason to commend a cautious approach. It is important, however, that this reticence is healthy and not arising from a lack of knowledge or appropriate clinical training. The head and neck nurse needs to be fully conversant with a wide range of techniques – from emergency tracheostomy to the much less acute situations such as arranging the best type of speaking device for the long-term laryngectomee. In this chapter we will deal with the issues with which the nurse is most likely to be involved in the ward situation. It is beyond the remit of the book to discuss advanced life support and respiratory management, which is more the domain of intensive care, and is adequately covered elsewhere.

## ANATOMY AND PHYSIOLOGY

The upper airway includes the nasal and oral cavities, pharynx and larynx. Functionally, the arrangement of the upper airway is not ideal. Food must pass the upper airway in order to reach the oesophagus. The pharynx, therefore, has two conflicting functions: it must rapidly constrict during swallowing, yet maintain patency during inspiration. Breathing and speech must be interrupted during a swallow.

The anatomy and physiology of each of these organs, apart from the nose, is dealt with elsewhere in this book, so here we will only deal with the nasal cavity.

## The nose

The nose consists of the external nose and the nasal cavity, which is divided into right and left halves by the midline nasal septum. The nasal cavity extends from the nostrils to the posterior end of the nasal septum. Each half of the cavity has olfactory, vestibular and respiratory parts depending on the type of epithelial covering.

Most of the cavity is the respiratory area, lined with the pseudostratified ciliated columnar epithelium of a very vascular mucosa, the function of which is to warm, humidify and filter inspired air. The vestibular area is the region just inside the nostril, a centimetre or so in depth, lined by skin which is continuous with the skin of the face. The olfactory area occupies the roof and uppermost parts of the nasal septum and lateral wall, over but not below the superior concha.

### The external nose

This is the part of the nose that projects from the face. It consists of the nasal bones (the bridge), the lateral (upper) and greater (alar or lower) cartilages. It is supported in the midline by the cartilaginous part of the nasal septum. A pad of fibrofatty tissue forms the lateral boundary of the nostril; this and the adjacent cartilage are moved by the compressor and dilator nares muscles.

### The nasal cavity

The nasal cavity is divided into two irregular parts by a central septum. The posterior bony part of the septum is formed by the perpendicular plate

of the ethmoid bone and the vomer. Anteriorly, it consists of hyaline cartilage (Fig. 2.1). In cross-section the cavity is pear-shaped, but the conchae
project into it with increasing prominence from above down (Fig. 2.2).

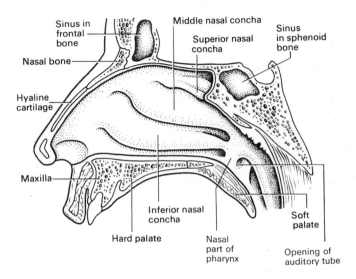

**Figure 2.1**    Lateral wall of nasal cavity. From Wilson & Waugh 1996, with permission.

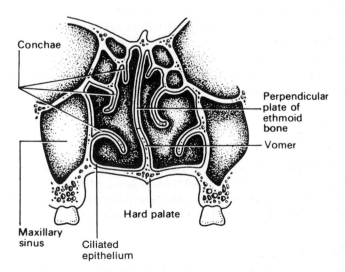

**Figure 2.2**    Interior of the nose viewed from the front. From Wilson & Waugh 1996, with
permission.

The roof is formed by the cribriform plate of the ethmoid bone, the sphenoid, frontal and nasal bones. The floor is formed by the roof of the mouth and consists of the hard palate in front and the soft palate behind. The hard palate is composed of the maxilla and palatine bones.

There are important openings into the nasal cavity from the paranasal sinuses: the maxillary sinuses in the lateral walls, the frontal and sphenoidal sinuses in the roof, and the ethmoidal sinuses in the upper part of the lateral walls. The nasolacrymal ducts, which drain tears from the eyes, also open into the lateral walls.

## The lateral wall of the nasal cavity

The lateral wall is semicircular in shape, sloping from the broad nasal floor to the narrow roof. Three nasal conchae (turbinate bones) project downwards like scrolls from the wall. Beneath the free inferior border of each is a space, called the superior, middle and inferior meatus, respectively. Above the superior concha is the sphenoethmoidal recess. The sphenoidal sinus opens into this recess, and the posterior ethmoidal air cells open into the superior meatus. The nasolacrimal duct opens into the inferior meatus. The middle meatus receives all the other openings into the lateral wall.

The blood supply and nerve supply of the lateral wall almost coincide. If the wall can be divided into four quadrants the supply can be described as follows.

**Posterosuperior quadrant.** This is supplied by the lateral posterior superior nasal vessels and nerves from the maxillary artery and the pterygopalatine ganglion. Both reach the lateral wall by passing through the sphenopalatine foramen.

**Posteroinferior quadrant.** This is supplied by branches of the greater palatine artery and posterior inferior nasal nerve.

**Anterosuperior quadrant.** This is supplied by the anterior ethmoidal nerve, which passes down through the cribriform plates. The nerve gives off these lateral branches as well as septal branches, and passes out to the surface, where it is called the external nasal nerve.

**Anteroinferior quadrant.** This is supplied by the anterior superior alveolar nerve on its way to its termination in the tiny septal branch. The arteries, on the other hand, are assisted by the alar branch of the superior labial and perforating branches of the greater palatine arteries.

The venous drainage from the central parts of the wall is via veins accompanying the arteries into the pterygoid plexus. Posteriorly the veins go to the pharyngeal plexus, while anteriorly they pass to the facial vein. The lymphatic drainage follows that of the veins.

## The nasal septum

The nasal septum consists of two bones – the vomer and the ethmoid – and a cartilage which extends forwards to give shape and prominence to the nose.

The nerve and blood supply to the septum are similar. The nasopalatine nerve and the sphenopalatine artery and the medial posterior superior nasal branches supply the posterior and inferior parts of the septum. The anterosuperior part is innervated by the septal branches of the anterior ethmoidal nerve, with the olfactory part also receiving olfactory nerve filaments. The anterior ethmoidal artery is assisted by branches that enter the anterior nares from the superior labial branch of the facial artery.

Venous drainage of the septum is towards the face from the front half and with the sphenopalatine artery from the back half, the blood flowing into the pterygoid plexus or via ethmoidal veins reaching the ophthalmic or inferior cerebral vessels.

Lymph drainage from the front half of the septum is into the submandibular nodes and from the posterior part to retropharyngeal and anterosuperior deep cervical nodes.

## ASSESSMENT

### History

As with any clinical assessment evaluation of the airway begins with the taking of a thorough history as this determines the course of further investigations. The timing, frequency, severity and character of symptoms and their association with other symptoms need to be noted. The main symptoms of upper airway dysfunction are the following.

• *Stridor.* This is the harsh sound produced by turbulent airflow through the upper airway. Typically, inspiratory stridor is characteristic of an extrathoracic lesion and expiratory stridor of an intrathoracic lesion. Stridor on breathing in and out is present with more critical lesions anywhere in the upper airway.

• *Cough.* Cough is considered pathological when it occurs with increased frequency or when it is productive. If it is consistently associated with swallowing, it may indicate aspiration, when it is usually associated with a lesion that prevents closure of the larynx or obstructs the upper digestive tract with resultant spillage into the airway.

• *Hoarseness.* Even the smallest true vocal cord lesion can produce alterations in voice. Constant progressive hoarseness often indicates a more serious disease such as laryngeal carcinoma. Intermittent hoarseness is usually associated with more benign problems such as vocal abuse or secondary to postnasal drip.

Other symptoms of upper airway disease include dysphagia (difficulty in swallowing) and odynophagia (pain on swallowing), haemoptysis, referred otalgia and the globus phenomenon (the sensation of a lump in the throat).

# Examination

The patient with upper airway dysfunction should undergo a complete head and neck examination, chest auscultation and neurological examination. It must be remembered that the patient with upper airway disease may also have lower respiratory tract disease, and the actual cause of symptoms may be difficult to distinguish.

Physical examination of areas above the pharynx is dealt with elsewhere, so here we will deal only with the structures below it.

The larynx, hypopharynx and the nasopharynx can be evaluated with a mirror in most cases. The rigid 90° telescope is a useful alternative. Flexible nasolaryngoscopy can be used in patients with a sensitive gag reflex and is helpful in patients with neurological problems since it does not interfere with pharyngeal or laryngeal function.

## Physiological testing

Common physiological testing for upper respiratory tract disease includes polysomnography, pulmonary function tests, laryngeal and pharyngeal electromyography and a number of phonatory tests.

## Imaging

**Plain radiography.** Lateral and anteroposterior plain radiographs are often used as screening examinations for patients with airway compromise. They are useful in evaluating diseases that produce deviation or narrowing of the airway as well as detecting foreign bodies within the airway. Chest views are also helpful in that they show mediastinal masses, parenchymal masses, infiltrates, pneumothoraces and effusions.

**Fluoroscopy.** This is useful for the confirmation of plain radiographs.

**Ultrasonography.** Ultrasonography is limited in the assessment of the airway, because of the sonographic barrier that air produces. It is most useful in the evaluation of solid or cystic extrinsic cervical airway masses.

**Arteriography.** Anomalies of the great vessels and vascular masses can be studied using arteriography, but increasingly CT scanning with intravenous contrast and MRI are being used as non-invasive alternatives.

**Computed tomography.** High resolution CT scanning can produce images of the most intricate structures in the head and neck. It can provide cross-sectional views in the axial plane for the neck (Fig. 2.3) and in the axial and coronal planes for head and face scanning (Fig. 2.4). Spatial delineation is excellent, and bony definition is superior to all other imaging modalities. Unfortunately, it is costly, involves high radiation exposure and is limited to axial scans for the larynx and trachea.

**Magnetic resonance imaging.** MRI has many of the advantages of CT scanning in terms of the views obtainable but does not rely on ionising

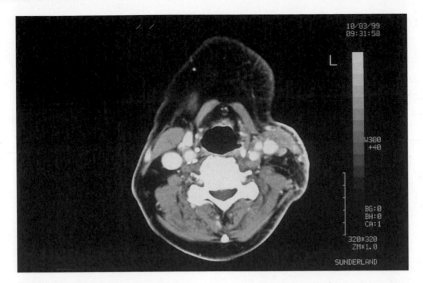

**Figure 2.3** Axial CT scan of neck.

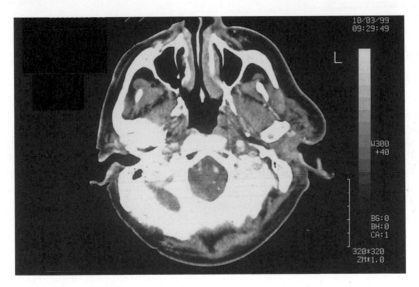

**Figure 2.4** Axial CT scan of head.

radiation and can demonstrate an anatomical site in multiple views although bone is not seen (Fig. 2.5).

## Endoscopic assessment

Sophisticated technology now allows excellent visualisation of the airways for both diagnostic and therapeutic purposes. In general, flexible scopes

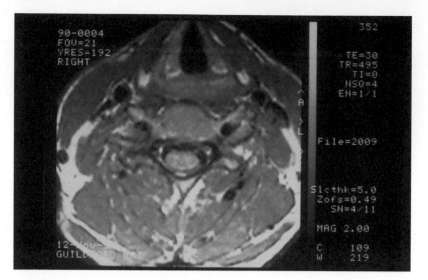

**Figure 2.5**   Axial MRI scan of neck.

can be used under topical anaesthesia with greater patient comfort than their rigid counterparts. Furthermore, they interfere less with function, but they are less useful for surgical intervention.

## PLANNING

Airway obstruction can be acute or chronic in nature. In acute airway obstruction the individual will have difficulty maintaining adequate levels of oxygenation; whereas, in subacute airway obstruction, respiratory difficulty often progresses over days and hypercapnia with or without hypoxia develops.

Hypercapnia can lead to acidosis and mental obtundation that complicates management. In chronic airway obstruction, the respiratory problem develops gradually, and patients do not usually have difficulty with either hypoxaemia or hypercapnia at rest. Progression of the obstruction or concurrent medical illness, however, may stimulate the development of subacute airway obstruction.

There are many causes of airway obstruction, and clearly the planning of nursing intervention is dependent on the basic aetiology of the problem The causes are listed in Box 2.1.

## IMPLEMENTATION

It is not our intention here to deal in detail with the routine management of all the causes of airway obstruction. We will discuss only those that have a

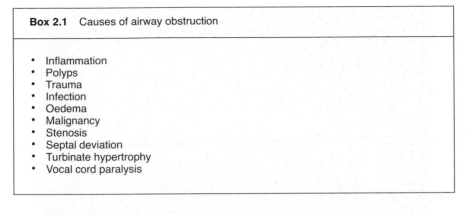

Box 2.1   Causes of airway obstruction

- Inflammation
- Polyps
- Trauma
- Infection
- Oedema
- Malignancy
- Stenosis
- Septal deviation
- Turbinate hypertrophy
- Vocal cord paralysis

significant nursing input, although we recognise that, with the increasing responsibilities of Clinical Nurse Specialists, the scope of nursing involvement may be different in various clinical settings and, indeed, with time.

## Management of acute airway problems

When inadequate oxygenation is recognised postoperatively the cause can usually be attributed to either surgical or anaesthetic complications or to the underlying disease process. It is important, however, to remember that the principles of airway management remain the same whatever the aetiology. The simple application of the ABC of the resuscitation procedure will save many more lives than inappropriately administered advanced techniques.

Impairment of the airway may be due to lack of muscle tone but more commonly it is due to obstruction with secretions or foreign material such as food or vomit. In the conscious patient the Heimlich manoeuvre is useful, but if unconsciousness has occurred then digital examination and laryngoscopic inspection are indicated before the swift establishment of an airway.

In many cases an adequate airway can be gained with simple measures such as the jaw thrust with extension of the neck, and that is all that may be required until the patient takes control of his or her own breathing. If the history is that of trauma then clearly the neck must not be extended but should be stabilised in the midline and a suitable airway introduced. Needless to say, appropriately maintained equipment such as suction apparatus, Magill forceps, laryngoscopes and a good range of airway devices is mandatory. The commoner airway devices are briefly mentioned below.

**Oropharyngeal airways.** The Guedel airway (Fig. 2.6) is a very effective device but still needs supplementary jaw support. An appropriate size needs to be selected from the colour-coded range and inserted curve

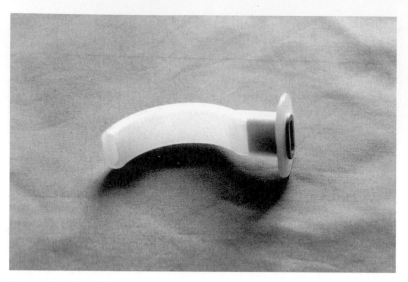

**Figure 2.6**   Guedel airway.

upwards into the vault of the palate before turning it over so that the tip points down towards the pharynx. Most modern types have an inner strengthener of reinforced plastic to resist biting forces, which may occlude the airway itself.

**Barrier and shield devices.** Most of these devices comprise a plastic sheet with a central airway that incorporates a one-way patency valve (Fig. 2.7). They are compact and inexpensive but are difficult to seal effectively around the contours of the face, particularly in edentulous patients.

**Ventilation masks.** Ventilation masks (Fig. 2.8) are produced in a range of sizes, and it is essential that a suitable size for the patient is used to achieve an effective seal. They are usually compatible with the tubing used to deliver oxygen to the patient; with a reservoir bag the patient can be ventilated until a stable airway is established.

### Endotracheal intubation

In most centres this procedure is carried out by suitably trained medical staff, although in the emergency situation this may not be the case. Oral intubation with the correctly sized cuffed tube is the method of choice, but, if the oral structures are badly damaged as a result of trauma, nasal intubation may be required. Nasal intubation, however, should not be attempted where midface injuries are present, as cases have been reported of tubes being misguided into the cranium.

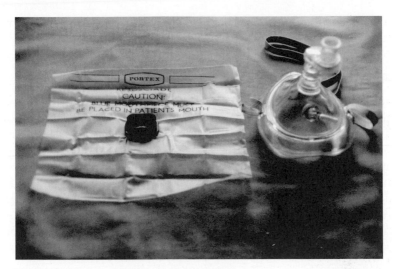

**Figure 2.7**   Barrier and shield devices.

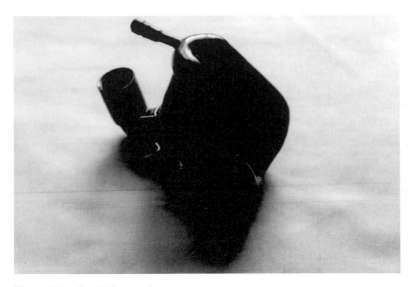

**Figure 2.8**   Ventilation mask.

## Tracheostomy

Fortunately, nowadays, this is rarely carried out as an emergency procedure. Cricothyroid access may be lifesaving in situations where the extent of damage is so great that intubation of the airway is not possible by other means, but formal tracheostomy should be performed as an elective procedure by an experienced surgeon in order to minimise the associated complications. This will be discussed more fully later in this chapter.

## Nasal obstruction

The treatment of nasal obstruction is determined by the findings of the history, physical examination and investigations carried out. Treatment can be divided broadly into medical, surgical and other, although a combination may occasionally be necessary.

Nasal surgery may involve the placement of nasal packs for a period of time after surgery. It is therefore important for the nurse to be familiar with the differing types of packs available and the correct method of their removal. Frequently, following removal of the nasal packs, a short brisk episode of bleeding can occur which usually settles spontaneously.

### Medical management

Medical management of nasal obstruction can involve one or more treatment options:

- elimination of the underlying irritant
- topical vasoconstrictors (short term)
- steroids (systemic preparation, injection locally, or topical aerosols)
- antihistamines
- antibiotics
- topical preparations
- cromolyn sodium
- analgesics
- diuretics
- anticholinergics
- allergy workup and elimination of the allergin or immunotherapy.

### Surgical management

This may involve:

- septal surgery consisting of submucous resection or septoplasty
- septal surgery inclusive of external deformity, septal rhinoplasty
- turbinate surgery consisting of submucous resection or partial turbinectomy
- chemical cauterisation, electrocautery or cryosurgery for mucosal disease
- surgical debulking or removal of neoplasms or granulomatous disease.

# Epistaxis

Although nasal haemorrhage is rarely life threatening, fatal consequences resulting from spontaneous nasal haemorrhage have been reported. These have included aspiration, hypotension, and hypoxia with resultant myocardial infarction.

In 10% of cases the aetiology of epistaxis is unknown. The aetiology, however, can be the result of multiple factors, each playing a minor role (Box 2.2). The management of epistaxis is affected by the following factors:

- degree of haemorrhage
- site of epistaxis
- patient age
- history of precipitating factors (trauma or surgery)
- prior history of bleeding
- complicating medical conditions
- use of medication that alters coagulation
- patient's general health.

In addition, treatment of epistaxis can involve the following:

- cauterisation
- embolisation
- cryotherapy
- nasal packing
- endoscopic cauterisation
- surgical reconstruction
- laser photocoagulation
- surgery
- greater palatine foramen block.

Within the field of head and neck nursing the main areas of treatment in which nursing staff will be involved include superficial cauterisation of the blood vessels in the Little's area and nasal packing. Nasal packing can be anterior or posterior. Several differing types of nasal packing are available, and choice may be based on clinician's preference. Anterior packs remain

---

**Box 2.2**    Aetiology of epistaxis

- Hypertension
- Nasal trauma
- Anticoagulant drugs
- Blood dyscrasias
- Atrophic rhinitis
- Malignancy

in situ for 24–48 hours. Posterior packs are generally used when, although adequate placement of anterior packs has occurred, bleeding persists. Placement of a posterior pack usually requires the placement of an anterior pack for stabilisation; posterior packs are generally left in situ for 3–5 days.

Nursing management of the individual with nasal packs in situ will involve maintenance of oral hygiene. In addition, particularly with posterior packs, all patients will experience difficulty in swallowing; therefore, maintenance of body fluids is of vital importance. Management also involves bed rest whilst the packs are in situ; therefore, deep vein thrombosis is of particular concern, and the use of elastic stockings is advocated.

## Tracheostomy

Although the ultimate goal in managing upper airway obstruction is to avoid tracheostomy, this procedure is indicated for those individuals who refuse other interventions, who have not had success with other techniques, or who represent a poor medical risk. The purpose of a tracheostomy is to bypass the airway obstruction and to maintain phonation and deglutition (Wanamaker & Eliachar 1995). A tracheostomy is sometimes performed when major intraoral resection and bilateral neck dissections are proposed and massive swelling is anticipated which may compromise the airway.

There are two basic techniques for forming a tracheostomy. These are the standard surgical tracheostomy (SST) and the percutaneous tracheostomy (PCT). Powell et al (1998) suggest that the development of PCT is based on the number and frequency of complications for the standard technique. These include postoperative haemorrhage, pneumothorax, tracheal fistulae, tube occlusion, tube displacement and subcutaneous emphysema. In addition they report frequent aspiration difficulties leading to pneumonia.

The upper respiratory tract is responsible for warming, moistening and filtering inhaled air. When a tracheostomy is performed, the upper airway is bypassed and these protective mechanisms are lost. Inhalation of dry air increases the risk of chest infection as a result of blockage of the tube with mucus due to paralysis of the cilia and drying of the mucus. An artificial means of humidification is therefore required during the immediate postoperative phase. Initially the tube causes irritation of the trachea, thus increasing mucosal secretion. Frequent suction may thus be required at this stage. Hooper (1996) suggests, however, that suction should only be performed as the individual requires it, rather than routinely. The removal and cleaning of the inner tracheostomy tube also reduces the tendency of the tube to obstruct.

If the individual develops respiratory distress the following procedures need to be adopted.

- Establish upright position of the individual, remove inner tube if blocked, clean as recommended by manufacturer and replace.
- If inner tube is not blocked and respiratory distress persists, then proceed to suction.
- If respiratory distress persists, the tracheostomy tube needs to be changed.

It is very important for nursing staff to remain calm when dealing with this situation, in order to relieve the patient's anxiety and reduce bodily movements which lead to the tube stimulating the cough reflex.

There are several types of tracheostomy tube commercially available but the basic types are: low pressure cuffed (Fig. 2.9a) and non-cuffed tubes (Fig. 2.9b) (the cuff of the tube providing added protection to the lower airway), fenestrated and non-fenestrated (Fig. 2.9c) (the fenestration allowing improved phonation).

Initially it can be very difficult for the individual to become accustomed to expectorating through the tracheostomy tube, and encouragement and education may need to be maintained until competence is achieved. The initial tracheostomy tube placed will consist of a cuffed tube in order to protect the airway during the initial 24 hours. It is important to remember that whilst the cuff is inflated the patient is unable to speak and therefore an alternative means of communication will be required. Moreover, during this period the individual may have discomfort and/or difficulty in swallowing, because of pressure from the cuff. The cuff is generally deflated 24 hours after surgery, and as there are often secretions lying above the cuff, which may become displaced when the cuff is deflated, it is important for the patient to cough and expectorate in order to clear them. Following deflation of the cuff the individual can, by occluding the tracheostomy tube with a thumb, vocalise. Speech can be improved by the placement of a fenestrated tracheostomy tube which allows increased airflow to the vocal cords.

Changing of the first tracheostomy tube is generally on the fifth postoperative day, by which time a well-defined tract has developed which makes tube changing easier. The first change of the tracheostomy tube should be carried out by a very experienced member of the team. The essential equipment is shown in Figure 2.10.

Whilst the tracheostomy tube is in place, physiotherapy for breathing and coughing is an essential part of the patient's treatment, for the ability of the individual to expectorate independently will minimise the need for tracheal suction. Within the early postoperative phase, tracheal suction is necessary to maintain a clear airway. As sensations such as choking, breathlessness and pain are associated with this procedure, again it is best carried out by an experienced team member, but eventually the individual and home carers can be educated to perform this procedure, thus promoting independence and control.

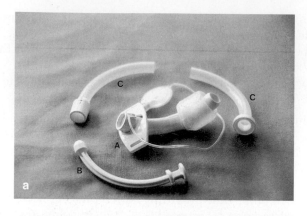

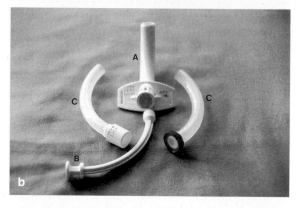

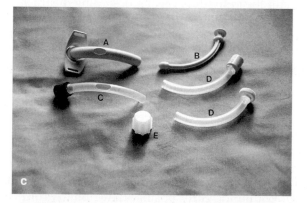

**Figure 2.9** Tracheostomy tubes: (a) Cuffed: A, outer cannulae; B, introducer; C, inner cannulae. (b) Non-cuffed: A, cuffed outer cannulae; B, introducer; C, inner cannulae. (c) Fenestrated and non-fenestrated: A, fenestrated outer cannulae; B, introducer; C, fenestrated inner cannulae; D, non-fenestrated inner cannulae; E, decannulation plug.

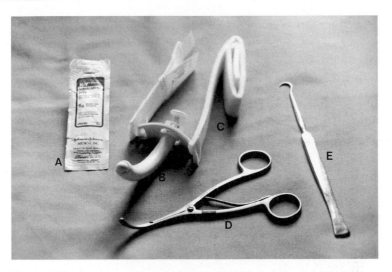

**Figure 2.10**  Equipment for changing a tracheostomy tube: A, lubricating gel; B, tracheostomy tube; C, Dale tracheostomy tube holders; D, tracheal dilator; E, tracheal hook.

In situations where the need for a tracheostomy is permanent, the management should where possible be established with the patient. This should include removal, cleaning and replacement of the inner tube, stoma care and renewing of the tracheostomy tube. Clearly, more support from relatives or a Community Nurse is required if the patient is unable to manage because of physical or mental impairment.

## EVALUATION

In some situations the evaluation of airway management needs to be almost instantaneous. It goes without saying that, for example, if a victim of severe facial trauma cannot be suitably intubated then a transtracheal approach is indicated immediately. Most of the time, however, we can evaluate our care at a more leisurely pace!

From a nursing point of view, much evaluation will concentrate on the factors which affect the patient's comfort and overall wellbeing. As well as ensuring an unobstructed airway, we need to maximise the patient's ability to communicate effectively, to remain infection-free and to manage a suitable oral intake. These considerations will be discussed in the relevant chapters, but it is important to remember that most of them are intricately related to the airway.

REFERENCES

Hooper M 1996 Nursing care of the patient with a tracheostomy. Nursing Standard 10(34): 40–43
Powell D M, Price P D, Forrest A 1998 Review of percutaneous tracheostomy. The Laryngoscope 108: 170–177
Wanamaker J R, Eliachar I 1995 An overview of treatment options for lower airway obstruction. Coleman J A, Duncauge J A (eds) The Otolaryngologic Clinics of North America 28(4), W B Saunders, London
Wilson K J W, Waugh A 1996 The respiratory system. In: Ross and Wilson's Anatomy and physiology in health and illness, 8th edn. Churchill Livingstone, New York

# 3

# Mouth care

'Bid them wash their faces,
And keep their teeth clean'

(Shakespeare – *Coriolanus*, Act II)

KEY POINTS

- Mouth care – who does it?
- The microbiological basis of oral problems
- Aids to assessment and treatment
- Specific mouth care problems in head and neck patients
- Multidisciplinary mouth care

## INTRODUCTION

The mouth is a complex structure which carries out a number of complicated functions important to us all. Life becomes much less pleasurable if the mouth is not working well, and most of us recognise the value of keeping it clean and healthy. We feel and look better, we have more confidence in close social contact and we enjoy all the sensations of eating and drinking to the full. Everyone should be encouraged to take effective oral hygiene measures each day and to have regular dental treatment. Mouth care is part of the total nursing care of all patients, whether they be admitted under the general surgeons, the haematologists or the orthopaedic surgeons.

Most patients are, quite rightly, left to look after their own oral hygiene, but the nursing assessment should include an intraoral inspection and a recognition of any obvious deficiencies. Some patients are totally unable to look after their mouths – for example, the unconscious and those on ventilators – and nurses should pay as much attention to this part of care as they would to other areas of nursing care. Other patients – for example, the mentally or physically handicapped and some children – may require a variable degree of nursing assistance.

Patients undergoing surgery involving the mouth, jaws and pharynx, or having pathology in these areas must have meticulous mouth care. This involves patient education, practical instruction and possibly supervision by a variety of health care workers. Nurses have an important role to play in all these areas. The orthopaedic patient recovering from an operation to fix a fracture of the tibia is not to be expected to, and indeed would be actively discouraged from, pouring the contents of the dinner plate over the wound! But this is exactly what is required of the patient who has just undergone open reduction and fixation of a fracture of the mandible! Of course the blood supply of the mouth is better than that of the lower leg and healing may be less of a problem, but the same complications will arise if the intraoral wound and its environment are not kept clean (despite taking a soft or sloppy diet). Unfortunately, mouth care is frequently overlooked or even deliberately ignored by both patients and nurses. On the head and neck ward it is clearly high on the list of priorities and the nursing staff are ideally suited to advise and encourage a similar attitude in their colleagues in high dependency areas as well as on the general medical, surgical and paediatric wards.

## ANATOMY AND PHYSIOLOGY

As in most other clinical areas effective head and neck nursing is based on a sound knowledge of the basic medical sciences. This is nowhere more apparent than in the care of the oral cavity both in health and disease. The close adaptation of structure to function in the mouth, combined with the dynamic microbial environment, makes this a fascinating area of nursing care.

The mouth extends from the lips to the palatoglossal arches. It is enclosed by the lips and cheeks. The space between these structures and the teeth and gingivae is the vestibule. The space inside the dental arches is the mouth cavity proper. The floor of this cavity is occupied by the tongue, and the roof is the hard palate. Posteriorly it is bounded by the soft palate.

The mouth is for eating and speaking as well as serving as an emergency airway in dyspnoea. The lips are essential for speech and are used to grasp food and suck liquids. The vestibule accommodates food, and the buccinator muscle returns it to the molars for chewing.

The tongue also grasps food, moves it around the mouth and has a role in swallowing. Fine movements of the tongue are used in speech and it plays a major part in detecting texture and taste.

The oral cavity is lined with mucous membrane which is adherent to the deeper structures and covered in stratified squamous epithelium.

## The teeth

At birth all the teeth are present in an immature form in the maxilla and the mandible. They then erupt in two phases which overlap – the deciduous dentition or 'baby teeth' and the permanent dentition. The normal times of eruption are shown in Table 3.1.

The shapes of the different teeth and the basic structure are shown in Figures 3.1 and 3.2.

**Table 3.1**  The times of eruption and notation of teeth

| Deciduous teeth | | Notation |
|---|---|---|
| 6 months | Lower central incisors | A |
| 7 months | Upper central incisors | A |
| 8 months | Upper lateral incisors | B |
| 9 months | Lower lateral incisors | B |
| 1 year | First molars | D |
| 18 months | Canines | C |
| 2 years | Second molars | E |
| Permanent teeth | | |
| 6 years | First permanent molars | 6 |
| 7 years | Central incisors | 1 |
| 8 years | Lateral incisors | 2 |
| 9 years | First premolars | 4 |
| 10 years | Second premolars | 5 |
| 11 years | Canines | 3 |
| 12 years | Second permanent molars | 7 |
| 18 years + | Third permanent molars | 8 |

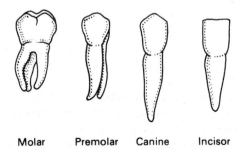

Molar      Premolar      Canine      Incisor

**Figure 3.1**  The shapes of the permanent teeth. From Wilson & Waugh 1996, with permission.

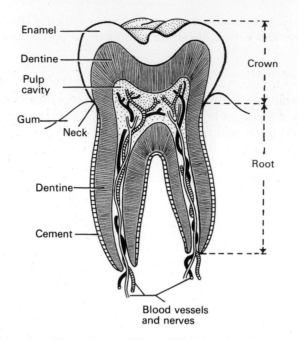

Enamel

Dentine

Pulp
cavity

Gum

Neck

Crown

Root

Dentine

Cement

Blood vessels
and nerves

**Figure 3.2**   A section of a tooth. From Wilson & Waugh 1996, with permission.

Whilst the detailed morphology and composition of individual teeth are of interest to the restorative dental team, they are less relevant to this text. What is of paramount importance to the head and neck nurse, however, is the position of the teeth and how the upper and lower teeth meet together – the dental occlusion (Fig. 3.3)

The teeth are held in the alveoli or sockets on the ridges of the mandible and the maxilla by the periodontal membrane. The teeth in the upper jaw form a curve like a horseshoe. In the lower jaw the curve straightens out in the molar region. The upper teeth thus make a larger curve than the lower. The upper incisors lie in front of the lower when the teeth are in occlusion. The upper canine lies just behind the lower, in front of the first premolar and to their outer side. The palatal cusps of the upper premolars and molars lie in the groove between the lingual and buccal cusps of their opposite numbers. In this way each upper tooth articulates with its opposing tooth and the tooth behind it.

The innervation of the teeth is shown in Figure 3.4. In the upper jaw the molars are supplied by the dental branches of the posterior superior alveolar nerve. The anterior buccal root of the first molar is supplied by the middle superior alveolar nerve, which also supplies the two upper premolars. The canine and the incisors are supplied by the anterior superior alveolar nerve.

# Colour plate section

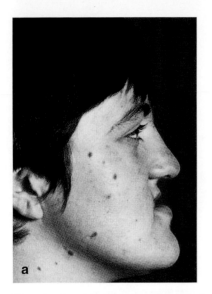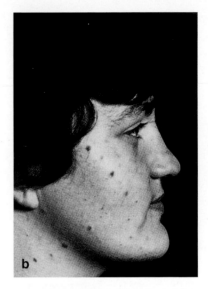

a
b

**Plate 1** A patient (a) before and (b) after bimaxillary surgery to correct her Class III skeletal jaw relationship.

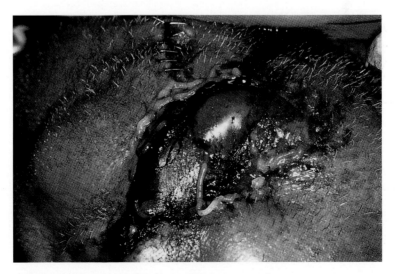

**Plate 2** A free flap showing signs of venous congestion.

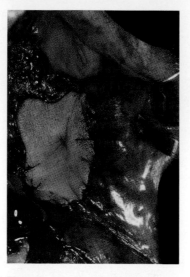

**Plate 3**   A well-perfused free flap.

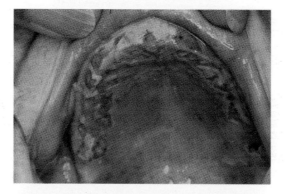

**Plate 4**   Acute pseudomembranous candidiasis.

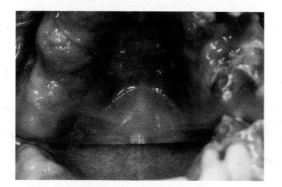

**Plate 5**   Acute atrophic candidiasis.

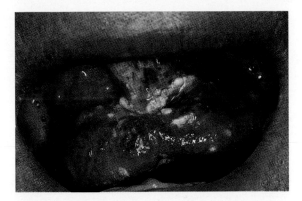

**Plate 6**  Speckled leucoplakia.

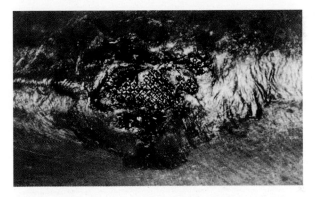

**Plate 7**  Black wound: necrotic; identified by presence of predominantly black or yellowish-brown tissue.

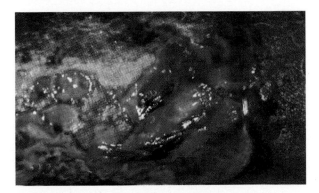

**Plate 8**  Yellow wound: sloughy; identified by formation of viscid, predominantly yellow layer of tissue.

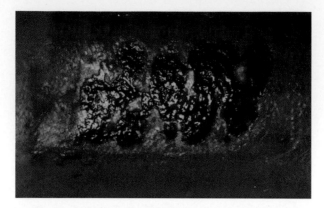

**Plate 9** Granulating wound: granular appearance; looks red and bleeds easily.

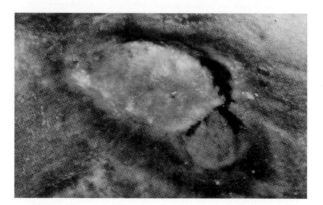

**Plate 10** Epithelialising wound: pink in appearance; tissue is very fragile and has to be kept moist.

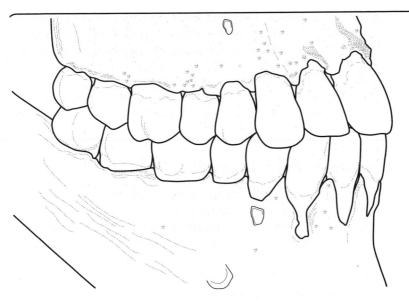

**Figure 3.3**   The ideal dental occlusion.

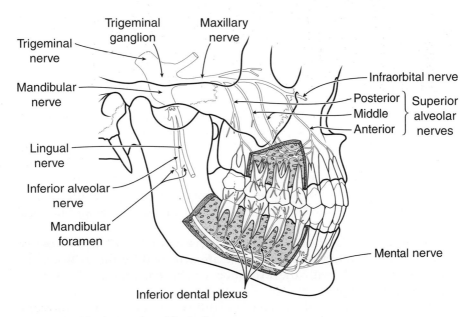

**Figure 3.4**   The innervation of the teeth.

In the mandible the premolars and molars receive their supply from the main trunk of the inferior alveolar nerve, whose terminal branch supplies the remaining teeth on the same side with some overlap to the central incisor on the opposite side.

The maxillary artery supplies blood to the upper teeth. It divides into branches that accompany the nerves and shares the same nomenclature. The lower teeth are supplied by the inferior alveolar artery from the maxillary artery.

## The musculature of the oral cavity

The muscles of the lips and cheeks are made up of some of the muscles of facial expression which are discussed in Chapter 7.

The main muscle of the floor of the mouth is the mylohyoid muscle. It arises from the inner aspect of the mandible and inserts along the connective tissue which forms the mylohyoid raphe in the midline and on the hyoid bone. On its superior surface on either side of the midline are the geniohyoid muscles. Contraction of these muscles pulls the hyoid bone upwards and forward, tightening the floor of the mouth and thus providing support for the tongue.

The loose connective tissue lateral to the tongue and resting on the mylohyoid muscle contains the sublingual gland, the deep part of the submandibular gland and its duct as well as the blood vessels and nerves of the area. It is a significant area because dental abscesses not infrequently drain into it and can spread downward over the posterior free edge of the muscle into the anterior neck or into the retropharyngeal space, with dire consequences (see Ch. 2).

## The tongue

The importance of the tongue's role in the maintenance of oral hygiene cannot be overestimated. It is a powerful, mobile organ which is able to reach all the outer surfaces of the teeth, around the vestibule and across the palate to remove adherent foodstuffs, plaque and other undesirable surface coatings. Figure 3.5 shows the roughened character of the surface of the tongue created by the presence of papillae. This is another example of the adaptation of structure to function in the grasping of food and as an 'intraoral brush'.

The musculature of the tongue is summarised in Table 3.2. It is worthy of note that all the muscles of the tongue are activated by the XIIth cranial nerve (hypoglossal) with the exception of the palatoglossus, which is supplied by the vagus.

The sensory supply to the tongue is slightly more complicated, reflecting its development from three pharyngeal arches. The anterior two thirds, or

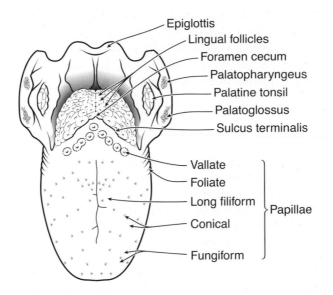

Epiglottis
Lingual follicles
Foramen cecum
Palatopharyngeus
Palatine tonsil
Palatoglossus
Sulcus terminalis

Vallate
Foliate
Long filiform
Conical
Fungiform
} Papillae

**Figure 3.5**  The surface of the tongue.

**Table 3.2**  The muscles of the tongue

| Classification | Muscle | Action | Innervation |
|---|---|---|---|
| Intrinsic | Vertical Horizontal Longitudinal | Curling, rolling and flattening the tongue | XII |
| Extrinsic | Styloglossus | Retrudes the tongue | XII |
| | Hyoglossus | Pulls the tongue down and back | XII |
| | Genioglossus | Posterior fibres protrude tongue, anterior fibres pull tip down | XII |
| | Palatoglossus | Pulls tongue and soft palate together | X |

presulcal part (but not the region of the vallate papillae) is supplied by the lingual nerve. The trigeminal component of this nerve mediates pain, temperature and touch, whilst the chorda tympani component mediates taste. The posterior third of the tongue is supplied by the IXth cranial nerve (glossopharyngeal) which has fibres for common sensation and taste.

The blood supply to the tongue is the lingual artery, and it is drained by the lingual vein into the internal jugular vein. It is the lymphatic drainage of the tongue, however, that has great clinical significance: there is considerable overlap across the midline. The tip is said to drain bilaterally to the submental nodes, and the remainder of the anterior part of the tongue drains to the submandibular nodes. The posterior part drains to the jugulo-omohyoid and other deep cervical nodes. Hence, all lymph from the tongue ultimately reaches the cervical nodes, but lymph (and of course associated tumour spread) from one side of the tongue can reach nodes on the opposite side of the neck.

## Salivary glands

Although the main salivary glands are bilateral extraoral structures, they secrete into the mouth. Their function is so crucial to oral health that they will be discussed in this chapter.

The largest salivary gland is the parotid gland, which is situated in front of the ear and behind the ramus of the mandible. The peripheral branches of the VIIth cranial nerve (facial) run through it. Its duct runs forward across the masseter muscle. At the anterior border of the muscle the duct turns inwards and opens into the oral vestibule in a papilla opposite the upper second molar. The gland secretes a serous saliva rich in amylase.

Next in size is the submandibular gland, which is situated in the posterior part of the floor of the mouth related to the medial aspect of the body of the mandible. Its duct runs forward and opens in the floor of the mouth as a small orifice lateral to the lingual fraenum. The saliva produced by this gland is mucinous.

The almond-shaped sublingual gland is situated in the floor of the mouth between the side of the tongue and the teeth. Its viscous saliva enters the mouth through a series of small ducts opening into a small sublingual fold.

In addition to these three sets of major salivary glands there are estimated to be between six hundred and a thousand minor salivary glands. These are small discrete masses occupying the submucosa throughout most of the oral cavity. They are not found, however, within the gingivae or in the anterior part of the hard palate. These glands are mucinous glands with the exception of the serous glands of von Ebner, which are found below the sulci of the circumvallate papillae and in the foliate papillae of the tongue.

## Saliva

Saliva is a very complex fluid produced by the salivary glands. Its contents are listed in Box 3.1 The functions of saliva include the following.

**Protection.**  Saliva provides a mechanical washing action which is particularly important in clearing sugars from the mouth (see 'Microbiology', below). Its glycoprotein content, which makes the saliva mucinous, forms a barrier for the mucosa against noxious stimuli, microbial toxins and minor

---

**Box 3.1**    The contents of saliva

---

- Proteins
    - Serum proteins
        - IgG
        - IgM
        - IgA
        - Albumin
        - $\alpha$ and $\beta$ globulins
    - Proteins produced within the glands
        - Factor VII
        - Factor IX
        - Factor VIII
        - Platelets factor
- Enzymes
    - Amylose
    - Lysozyme
    - Acid phosphatase
    - Cholinesterase
    - Lipose
    - Peroxidase
    - Kallikrein
- Mucoproteins
- Glycoproteins
- Blood group substances
- Hormones
- Carbohydrates
- Lipids
- Nitrogen-containing compounds
- Lactoferrin
- Inorganic substances
    - Sodium
    - Potassium
    - Chloride
    - Bicarbonate
    - Hydrogen ions
    - Iodine
    - Fluoride
    - Thiocyamate
    - Calcium
    - Phosphate

---

physical trauma. Calcium-binding proteins also occur in saliva; they help to form a salivary pellicle around the teeth, which may have a protective function.

**Buffering.** The buffering capacity of saliva is mainly due to its content of bicarbonate and phosphate ions. These are assisted by sialin, a peptide, and various other proteins. Many bacteria require specific pH conditions for maximal growth. The buffering capacity of saliva minimises the colonisation of pathogenic microbes by denying them a suitable pH. Furthermore, if acids produced from dietary sugars in the mouth by the bacteria in plaque are not rapidly buffered they begin to demineralise enamel and thus initiate dental caries.

**Digestion.** Saliva provides taste acuity, is used in food bolus formation, neutralises oesophageal contents, dilutes chyme and, because of its amylase content, breaks down starch.

**Taste.** Saliva is needed to dissolve substances to be tasted and to carry them to the taste buds. It also contains a protein called gustin which is thought to be necessary for the maturation of taste buds.

**Antimicrobial.** As well as the barrier and pH protection that saliva confers, it also has a range of proteins with other antimicrobial properties: lysozyme, for example, can hydrolyse the cell walls of some bacteria, and lactoferrin binds free iron, thus depriving the organisms of an essential element. Furthermore, there are antibodies present in saliva. The main one is IgA, which has the capacity to clump or agglutinate micro-organisms.

**Maintenance of teeth.** Saliva is saturated with calcium and phosphate ions which ensures that ionic exchange with the tooth surface is directed to the tooth. This is important in tooth maturation and enamel demineralisation.

**Tissue repair.** See Chapter 4.

## Microbiology

The oral cavity is a complex microbiological environment. It is colonised by many viruses, yeasts, protozoa and a wide range of bacterial species. Numerically bacteria dominate, and both Gram-positive and Gram-negative organisms are present.

The most prevalent oral streptococci belong to the species *S. mutans*, *S. sanguis*, *S. mitior*, *S. milleri* and *S. salivarius*. *S. mutans* is the most virulent and is implicated in dental caries. Many of the oral streptococci are opportunist pathogens, with *S. mitior* being commonly isolated from infective endocarditis and *S. milleri* from brain and liver abscesses.

The normal microbial flora of the mouth are associated with the two most prevalent infections known – dental caries and periodontal disease. Dental caries result from the localised dissolution of enamel by acid of microbial origin produced from the fermentation of dietary carbohydrates. Periodontal disease embraces several conditions, including gingivitis, acute ulcerative gingivitis, chronic and juvenile periodontitis, all of which attack the supporting tissues of the teeth. The common aetiological factor in dental caries and periodontal disease is dental plaque.

Dental plaque is a general term for the complex microbial community found on the tooth surface, embedded in a matrix of polymers of bacterial and salivary origin. Plaque that becomes calcified is referred to as calculus or 'tartar', and most oral hygiene measures are aimed at preventing its formation or facilitating the removal of plaque before it calcifies.

## ASSESSMENT

All diagnoses are dependent on a combination of history taking and examination, usually in that order. In this section, however, we will reverse the process and consider methods of inspecting the mouth before thinking about the main groups of patients treated by the head and neck specialties and the particular intraoral problems they may have.

## Examination of the mouth

The majority of doctors and nurses have no idea about how to inspect the mouth. They may catch a glimpse of a few teeth as they insert a tongue depressor, usually causing the patient to gag and retch, before asking 'Say, Ah!' and gazing momentarily at the soft palate! Indeed it has been shown that qualified nurses often lack the knowledge to assess oral hygiene and that mouth care is often provided by junior members of staff and not given high priority among nursing duties (Holmes & Mountain 1993).

Examining the mouth need not be difficult and should be methodical. It is important at the outset to explain the procedure to the patient and to be reassuring. The postoperative or trauma patient may have a sore mouth or jaw and be very apprehensive. A gentle, but thorough, technique is necessary. The minimal requirements are:

- patient and examiner in comfortable positions
- gloves
- a good light
- retractors.

*Positioning the patient*

The ideal place to position the patient is in a dental chair; it is specifically designed for this purpose, but it is not essential. The mouth can be examined quite adequately with the patient seated on a chair with a back support. If in bed, it is easier if the patient sits or lies back with the head supported by a pillow. The neck should be slightly extended; it is virtually impossible to carry out an intraoral examination with the chin on the chest. The examiner should also be in a comfortable position, not crouched or stooping over. The patient should be able to move the head easily at the request of the examiner to afford a better view of a particular part of the mouth.

*Universal precautions*

The examiner's hands and fingers are important pieces of equipment for carrying out a thorough inspection. Vision is important, but so is touch, and certainly performing mouth care requires contact with the intraoral tissues and hence the patient's saliva and possibly blood. Wearing adequately fitting gloves is essential when working within the mouth.

## Lighting

The examination should be carried out in a good ambient light, but this must be supplemented by a light source which can be directed into the mouth. This may be a torch, a headlight, an ENT head mirror or, better still, a static light which can be positioned by the examiner. If only a torch is available, a full examination and any mouth care procedures may require an assistant.

## Retractors

The lips, cheeks and tongue must be retracted by some means so that the whole mouth may be inspected. This can be done by the examiner's fingers, but it is often better, and kinder, to use retractors. The commonest, cheapest, but least effective is the wooden spatula tongue depressor. Dental mirrors can be used as well as a wide array of intraoral surgical instruments such as C-shape and Lacks retractors. Plastic cheek retractors are also available.

## Examination

The examination need not be difficult and should be methodical. Any dentures should be removed. After this the order doesn't really matter as long as all the areas of the mouth are inspected. It is, however, sensible to begin with the lips. Are they swollen, dry, cracked or ulcerated? What is their colour? Are there any lacerations or surgical wounds? Next, peel back the lips and look at the buccal and labial sulci, the reflections of the cheeks and lips. It is important to realise that it is not always helpful to have the mouth wide open. At this stage the inside of the cheeks can be seen. Look at the tongue and ask the patient to protrude it. Is it dry or coated? Lift the tongue up and inspect its ventral surface (most carcinomas of the tongue arise from the lateral border and the ventral surface, and this can be hidden from view), and take this opportunity to examine the floor of the mouth. Is saliva pooling here? Is the saliva good quality (thin and watery), or is it thick, stringy and mucinous? Look up at both the hard and soft palate. Is there a cleft or a maxillectomy cavity? Gently depress the tongue and examine the lateral aspect of the oropharynx and tonsils. Are they enlarged or is there an exudate? Get into a habit of examining the soft tissues in the same sequence. It is only when you know what a healthy mouth looks like that you will pick up abnormalities.

Look at the teeth and gums. Are they clean or covered by plaque, food debris or even calculus? Are they decayed or loose? Are any appliances fitted to the teeth or are the teeth wired or elasticated together? Are there any crowns or bridges? What do the gums look like – red, swollen? Inspect any dentures or obturators and see how they fit.

Having identified the essential components of the oral examination it would be useful to quantify our findings. Holmes & Mountain (1993) looked for a means of doing this and evaluated three different oral assessment guides. Although none of them proved ideal, the authors were able to compile a useful summary of the main components.

## Common findings in the oral examination

We have now considered the general principles of oral examination and the idea of an assessment tool. In what circumstances may we be required to apply them?

### Patients after surgery localised to the mouth

Perhaps the largest group are those patients having surgery carried out entirely within the mouth under local or general anaesthesia, as inpatients or outpatients. The surgery may be confined entirely to soft tissue or involve bone. It may be relatively simple surgery (although from the patient's point of view no surgery is simple), such as soft tissue biopsy or tooth extraction, or quite complex such as transposition of submandibular ducts. It matters little, as the problems posed are similar but to varying degrees. The point to stress is that any intraoral wound will cause the patient discomfort during eating, chewing, swallowing and certainly during mouth cleaning, and yet the mouth is grossly contaminated with micro-organisms and thus open to infection. A vicious circle ensues: the mouth is sore, if it is not kept clean it may become infected and cause further pain and delayed healing, and yet carrying out oral hygiene measures itself may cause discomfort. The teeth need to be clean and in good order before the surgery, and the patient should be made aware of the importance of maintaining good oral hygiene.

### Patients after surgery of the jaws

Patients undergoing surgery to the bones of the jaws, including removal of wisdom teeth, treatment of fractures, and osteotomies of the jaws, may have a number of extra problems. The first is that they may have limited jaw opening (trismus). This makes tooth brushing more difficult, and food debris is more likely to accumulate. Osteotomy patients may have orthodontic appliances or arch bars fixed to their teeth which collect debris and are difficult to clean. In addition the jaws may be wired or elasticated together, and this poses additional cleaning problems. The nurse must recognise these additional factors and plan to deal with them preoperatively.

### Patients following intraoral reconstructive surgery

Resection of intraoral tumours often requires reconstruction of the surgical defect with flaps. These may be quite simple and local, such as the nasolabial skin flap or the temporalis muscle flap. Pedicle flaps based on a defined vascular supply, for example the pectoralis myocutaneous flap, still have an important role to play but, because of its versatility, free tissue transfer using microvascular surgery is being used increasingly in reconstruction. The workhorse is still the fasciocutaneous radial forearm flap, but compound flaps comprising combinations of skin, muscle and bone – e.g. scapular and deep circumflex iliac artery (DCIA) flaps – are now used more frequently. The importance of careful postoperative nursing for the success of these procedures cannot be overstressed. Not only is the nurse required to maintain high quality intraoral wound care for these patients but the hour-to-hour monitoring of the flap condition is also firmly in the nursing remit, particularly in free flap surgery.

Care of the flap will be considered in Chapter 4, but here we will consider the monitoring aspect first. Occasionally it is possible to assess the blood flow to a flap with Doppler studies, but usually monitoring is based on clinical signs. Muscle flaps can be quite difficult to assess. They tend to be bulky and initially they ooze blood. A slough may form, and after a few days the flap 'pinks up' and epithelialises. A darkening of the flap colour is a bad sign and may require surgical intervention. Skin lined flaps, particularly in Caucasians, are easier to monitor. The important features are the colour, the capillary return, the temperature and the texture or consistency. A very pale white flap, particularly if it is cold, is very suggestive of failure of the arterial anastomosis. A dark, bluish appearance, perhaps slightly swollen or oedematous, indicates problems with the venous outflow (Plate 2). A healthy flap will be soft, warm and, in Caucasian skin, slightly pink (Plate 3). On compressing it gently it will blanch, and on removing the pressure it will immediately 'pink up'. An unhealthy flap will be firm or even hard, cool, swollen and the surface may blister. It will not blanch on pressure. Of course there are all 'shades of grey' in between, and it is only with frequent inspection that changes in the appearance can be detected. The important points to realise are that flaps can be resuscitated surgically if clinical signs of failure are picked up early, and that flaps may fail even if they have been well perfused for a few days. Perhaps the ultimate test to assess the vitality of a flap is to prick it with a sterile needle and see if it bleeds, how quickly it does so, and the colour of the blood. This test is best carried out by a senior member of the surgical team.

## Medically compromised patients

These patients can be considered in two groups, as follows.

**Patients whose conditions may produce pathology within the mouth.** This may cover a variety of groups, but examples are those who are immuno-suppressed for whatever reason and insulin dependent diabetics. They are more prone to opportunistic infections such as candida and may have delayed wound healing. Patients having had radiotherapy to the mouth and jaws also fall into this group. They will have xerostomia, which hastens dental caries, and predisposes them to candidiasis. Tooth extraction in this group may also lead to osteoradionecrosis, a painful and difficult condition to treat.

**Patients whose medical condition may be compromised by pathology or treatment within the mouth.** Good examples of these are patients with a history of rheumatic heart disease or those with prosthetic heart valves. Focal infection around the teeth or any surgical interference, for example tooth extraction, may produce a bacteraemia which in turn can result in a bacterial endocarditis. Despite modern antibiotic therapy this is still a life-threatening condition.

Antibiotic regimens and guidelines for prophylaxis vary from unit to unit. The essential requirements are well documented in the *British National Formulary* and its equivalent in the USA.

## Patients with malignant disease

Cancer patients are especially prone to oral problems resulting from the disease itself, chemotherapy or radiotherapy (Porter 1994). These problems are often exacerbated by a reduced oral intake due to general malaise and reduced motivation. The commonest problems are the following.

**Fungal infections.** Fungal infections in the mouth occur much more frequently in patients with advanced cancer than in the normal population, particularly in those receiving chemotherapy. Whilst chemotherapy is not a widely used choice of treatment for malignancies of the head and neck, patients are often referred to the specialty for treatment of oral complications of their therapy.

Clinically evident candidal infection is usually due to an opportunistic increase in the numbers of *Candida albicans* and its presentation is varied. Acute pseudomembranous candidiasis or 'thrush' (Plate 4) is generally associated with some local disturbance or systemic illness. It presents as a thick, white coating which can be wiped away to leave a red, raw and often bleeding base. If antibiotic or steroid is prolonged an acute atrophic candidosis may develop which presents as a red and painful area of mucosa, most commonly on the tongue.

Another common presentation is denture stomatitis (chronic atrophic candidiasis). It is characterised by erythema and oedema of the tissues directly under the denture (Plate 5). The continual wearing of ill-fitting dentures and poor denture hygiene are closely related aetiological factors. Angular cheilitis often occurs alongside denture stomatitis and shares the same causation: soreness, erythema and fissuring at the corners of the mouth. Deep folds of skin at the oral commissures allow pooling of saliva and tissue maceration.

Chronic hyperplastic candidiasis also arises at the corners of the mouth and may be more sinister. The lesions are seen as triangular, roughened areas of leucoplakia, often bilateral. These white plaques cannot easily be removed, and a number of them have red areas within them giving rise to the description of 'speckled leucoplakia' (Plate 6). They may be premalignant, particularly if associated with iron deficiency anaemia.

**Xerostomia.** The sensation of a dry mouth may be an age-related change or it may be a symptom of a recognised pathology such as Sjögren's syndrome (a combination of xerostomia, lack of tear secretion and an autoimmune disease such as rheumatoid arthritis). More commonly in the head and neck patient, however, it is an unpleasant fact that is usually either drug induced or the result of radiotherapy. Whatever the cause, it is a distressing condition, interfering with normal mastication, taste, swallowing and speech. In the dentate patient lack of saliva can lead to rampant dental caries, and in the edentulous patient denture retention is severely impaired. In both groups of patients the mucosa becomes dry and prone to ulceration and infection.

**Oral mucositis.** The cells in the oral mucosa proliferate rapidly and are very sensitive to both chemotherapy and radiotherapy. In the case of the former, ulceration is the prominent feature, and in the latter xerostomia, but the feature common to both is severe soreness which can be very distressing indeed.

**Ulceration.** There are many causes of oral ulceration (Box 3.2), and the differential diagnosis of the condition is beyond the remit of this text. It is worth making the general point, however, that oral ulceration may well represent a systemic problem which may coexist with or indeed be responsible for the local condition in the mouth.

# PLANNING

Planning of mouth care, as for other nursing care, is based on a comprehensive assessment and accurate nursing diagnosis. It is essential that this takes place at the earliest opportunity and preferably before any surgical intervention. Involvement of the patient, relatives and other members of the interdisciplinary team at this stage allows the nurse to devise a treatment plan that addresses the individual patient's needs. Furthermore, it allows some time to notify other members of the team who may need to be involved in treatment at a later stage, so that they can make any necessary baseline observations.

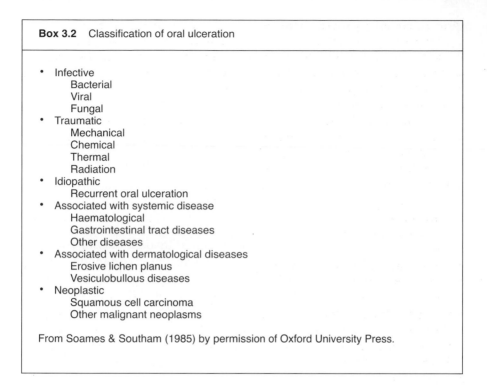

Box 3.2    Classification of oral ulceration

- Infective
    Bacterial
    Viral
    Fungal
- Traumatic
    Mechanical
    Chemical
    Thermal
    Radiation
- Idiopathic
    Recurrent oral ulceration
- Associated with systemic disease
    Haematological
    Gastrointestinal tract diseases
    Other diseases
- Associated with dermatological diseases
    Erosive lichen planus
    Vesiculobullous diseases
- Neoplastic
    Squamous cell carcinoma
    Other malignant neoplasms

From Soames & Southam (1985) by permission of Oxford University Press.

## IMPLEMENTATION

How do we as specialist nurses act on the information gained from the nursing diagnosis? How do we set about what is after all one of the most central roles of our discipline – the care of the mouth?

Hatton-Smith (1994) points out that this area of care is often seen by many nurses as a ritual based on the premise that 'this is the way it has always been done'. She highlights studies showing that some nurses are not fully familiar with the side effects, dilutions and expected results of oral health care products. Furthermore, she states that newly qualified nurses (who are often those detailed to this task) do not have the necessary knowledge to assess patients' oral requirements.

Needless to say, good nurse-administered mouth care must meet the individual patient's needs, and given the range of problems outlined in the previous section of this chapter the nurse must be flexible in approach. Rather than address individually each of the patient groups previously mentioned, we will now discuss the various treatments at our disposal and mention their applicability to individual problems.

## The aims of mouth care

The basic aims of mouth care are:

- achieve and maintain oral cleanliness
- prevent infection/stomatitis
- keep the oral mucosa moist
- promote patient comfort (Jenkins 1989).

How do we achieve these aims? Essentially, we need to consider the agents available to us and the means of getting them to the appropriate sites.

### Oral hygiene packs

Many hospitals supply their wards with an oral hygiene tray or pack, the contents of which are disposable or autoclavable. These commonly contain swabs or foam sticks to be used with whatever 'lotions and potions' may be at hand. Certainly they do not contribute to the idea of individualised care and interestingly may be more expensive and less effective than gentle tooth brushing (Harris 1980).

### Foam sticks

Foam sticks do have an important role in cleaning the oral mucosa and other tissues introduced to the oral cavity, such as free flaps and skin grafts, where the risk of trauma must be minimised. They do not remove the more adherent dental deposits. They are easy to use and carry a low risk of trauma.

### Moi-Stir® swabs

These are sticks with contoured cotton wool and impregnated with potassium chloride, sodium chloride, calcium chloride, magnesium chloride and sodium phosphate to make them moist. They have an unpleasant taste and are therefore only suitable for those who can tolerate the taste or who have no sense of taste.

### Toothbrushes

Research indicates that a toothbrush is the best way of cleaning teeth, and, as most patients are familiar with toothbrushing, it seems sensible to encourage it. The Bass method with a small-headed toothbrush is recognised as being the most effective way of removing plaque. The toothbrush is placed on the gingival margin at an angle of 45 degrees, and with very small vibratory movements the bristles of the brush will go subgingivally and collect the plaque.

## Interspace brush

This consists of a single-tufted brush with a pointed tip and is useful for patients with fitted orthodontic appliances after orthognathic surgery or those in intermaxillary fixation after trauma surgery.

## Interdental cleansing

This could involve the use of a dental floss or tape, wood sticks or special brushes for the removal of plaque between the teeth and for other areas that are inaccessible to normal brushing.

## Chlorhexidine gluconate products

In low concentrations chlorhexidine is bacteriostatic and in higher concentrations it is bacteriocidal. It is well recognised that it is effective in controlling plaque and oral candidiasis, making it an excellent aid to most mechanical cleansing methods. Commercially, chlorhexidine is available as solutions, gels and sprays, each of which has its own particular advantages.

**Solutions.** Chlorhexidine mouthrinse (0.2%) is used widely for its antimicrobial properties both to reduce plaque formation and in the treatment of oral infections. It can be used alone, being held in the mouth for several minutes, or applied to the tissues with sponges or swabs. Some patients, for example those having had third molars removed, find it beneficial to irrigate the sockets with chlorhexidine using a hypodermic syringe with an appropriate attachment such as a plastic quill. Stronger solutions can be useful to soak prostheses such as dentures, obturators or orthodontic appliances.

**Gels.** If the patient is unable to rinse normally, gels are a useful means of keeping the agent in contact with the tissues. For example they can be placed inside the dentures or inserted via an appropriate syringe into periodontal sockets in the management of periodontal disease.

**Sprays.** Chlorhexidine solutions if left in contact with the mucosa for prolonged periods may have a burning effect. In patients who are unable to cooperate – for example the ventilated patient – or in those where access is difficult, sprays may be particularly useful.

## Saline rinses

Probably the commonest recommendation to patients after minor oral surgical procedures is that of warm saline mouth baths. A teaspoonful of salt dissolved in a tumbler of warm water gives a cheap and effective means of keeping the surgical site clean and is alleged to promote healing.

### Sodium bicarbonate

Sodium bicarbonate (1% w/v) has mucosolvent properties and has been used to break down tenacious, viscous saliva. It has been used to debride crusted mouths as well as in toothpastes with the idea of neutralising plaque acids. There is little in the literature to support its use in the nursing context.

### Thymol

Thymol preparations are often combined with glycerine-based substances and may be used as a refreshing agent in oral hygiene regimes. It has no other function.

### Lemon and glycerine

These are used occasionally in some nursing settings, but their usefulness is questionable. Lemon may stimulate saliva flow but it can also irritate the inflamed or broken mucosa, and there are reports of a negative feedback loop operating leading to further inhibition of the salivary glands.

### Hydrogen peroxide

This is one of the most commonly used antiseptic solutions for mouth care despite the fact that it has been shown to delay wound healing in both animal and human wounds (Branemark & Ekholm 1967). Moreover, it is associated with significant mucosal abnormalities and is not very well accepted by patients (Tombes & Gallucci 1993).

## The management of specific problems in the mouth

### Xerostomia

The dry mouth is difficult to treat effectively. Often in very ill patients, medications and dosages are difficult to change, and radiation-damaged salivary tissue may be irreparable. Treatment is, therefore, symptomatic and largely dependent upon artificial salivas, of which there are a number available commercially. The two used most commonly in the UK are the murcin-based Saliva Orthana® (Nycomed, UK) and the carboxymethyl cellulose preparation Glandosane® (Fresenius Ltd). Both are available as sprays and the former as a lozenge. Neither product is medicated, although

Saliva Orthana® is fluoridated which may be an advantage in dentate. patients.

## Fungal infections

Whatever the predisposing factors to fungal infections the management is the same in terms of active treatment, although of course if the causative factor can be identified and removed the success of the therapy is greater. More specific measures must include increased oral hygiene measures to reduce secondary infection. For the dentate patient this may mean more effective and more frequent brushing and flossing. For the edentulous patient the care of dentures is of fundamental importance.

Daily cleansing and the rinsing of dentures after meals is, of course, essential. Ideally, they should be left out at night and soaked in a suitable disinfectant solution (Milton® (d) is commonly used for this purpose). Needless to say, the dentures need to be thoroughly rinsed before reinserting them into the mouth.

The maintenance or replacement of dentures is a more difficult problem. For many elderly people their dentures have become 'old friends' despite the fact that, due to weight loss and/or the resorption of the supporting oral tissues, they no longer fit and they give rise to several problems. Even if new dentures are made, the patient often rejects them and returns to the old set. Very often, simple measures such as easing over any hyperplastic tissue, cushioning over ulcers, and soft linings are more effective and can be carried out at the bedside if necessary.

Specific management of candidiasis requires antifungal medication. Topical agents such as nystatin or miconazole are available and can be placed inside the dentures where appropriate. Systemic antifungals, however, are often needed to completely eradicate the infection. The development of safer systemic drugs such as fluconazole (Diflucan®, Pfizer Ltd) and itraconazole (Sporanox®, Janssen Pharmaceuticals Ltd) has greatly facilitated therapy. The response is often rapid, thus allowing the infection to be brought under control before other dental treatment is carried out.

## Oral mucositis

The treatment of mucositis is aimed at reducing the discomfort. It is essential to work from the outside in, gently moistening and cleaning the lips and if necessary lubricating them before stretching them to gain access to the mouth. Benzyclamine hydrochloride 0.5% rinse (Difflam®, 3M Healthcare Ltd) is a good local anaesthetic agent. Once the mouth has been cleaned, application of an artificial saliva may be helpful. In severe cases this procedure should be repeated every 3–4 hours.

*Oral ulceration*

Treatment of oral ulceration is governed by the underlying cause. Some of the commonest causes are as follows.

**Bacterial.** Chlorhexidine rinses are mandatory, and in larger heavily infected ulcers tetracycline mouthrinses or the application of metronidazole gel may be effective, applied directly or packed with paraffin gauze.

**Viral.** Ulceration caused by the *Herpes simplex* virus must be treated promptly with acyclovir. Difflam® mouthrinse has proved helpful in easing the severe pain which often accompanies these infections.

**Inflammatory.** The discomfort that arises from inflammatory conditions of the mouth, which often presents as ulceration, such as aphthous lesions, erosive lichen planus, pemphigus and pemphigoid, is treated with corticosteroids. These are available as hydrocortisone lozenges (Corlan®, Evans) or as triamcinolone acetonide in an adhesive paste (Adcortyl in Orabase®, Squibb). If the condition is unresponsive to these or if the extent of the ulceration is preventing adequate oral intake of fluids, then prednisolone mouth rinse (5 mg in 10 mL of water qds) may be used. Systemic steroids are only justified in extreme cases.

## EVALUATION

It is clear from our discussion so far that there are a multiplicity of problems and possible solutions involved in the mouth care of the head and neck patient. Whatever the management, however, there is the ever present need to evaluate our actions rigorously. This audit needs to be repeated as often as is necessary and the treatment plan modified according to our findings. Moreover, any recorded changes can be used to educate and encourage the patient, who almost certainly needs every means of psychological support available.

The nurse occupies a key position within the multidisciplinary team of surgeons, dentists, dental hygienists, dieticians, prosthetists and the many others who may be involved, to coordinate and maximise the care delivered to the patient. All these professionals have different roles but these may overlap, and, as always, if this can be utilised positively the quality of care will be enhanced. For example, the dental hygienist, although usually based in an outpatient environment, can be of enormous help in looking after postoperative patients on the ward.

REFERENCES

Branemark P I, Ekholm R 1967 Tissue injury caused by wound disinfectants. Journal of Bone and Joint Surgery 49A: 48

Harris M 1980 Tools for mouthcare. Nursing Times 76: 340–342
Hatton-Smith C K 1994 A last bastion of ritualised practice? A review of nurses' knowledge of oral healthcare. Professional Nurse Feb: 304–308
Holmes S, Mountain E 1993 Assessment of oral status: evaluation of three assessment guides. Journal of Clinical Nursing 2(1): 35–40
Jenkins D A 1989 Oral care in the ICU: an important nursing role. Nursing Standard 4(7): 24–28
Porter H 1994 Mouth care in cancer. Nursing Times 90(14): 27–29
Soames J V, Southam J C 1985 Oral pathology. Oxford University Press, Oxford
Tombes M B, Gallucci B 1993 The effects of hydrogen peroxide rinses on the oral mucosa. Nursing Research 42(6): 332–336
Wilson K J W, Waugh A 1996 Ross and Wilson's Anatomy and physiology in health and illness, 8th edn. Churchill Livingstone, New York

# 4

# Wound care

'I dressed him and God healed him'

Ambroise Paré

---

KEY POINTS

- The dynamics of wound care
- Wound assessment techniques
- The care of intra- and extraoral wounds
- Agents: from tap water to leeches!

---

## INTRODUCTION

Nursing research has revolutionised the theory of wound management. It would seem, however, that the accumulated knowledge is not always applied in practice (Turner 1991). Some studies suggest that nurses may have a problem differentiating between pus and slough, whilst others reveal a lack of understanding of the healing process (Sutton 1989). Indeed as late as 1995 Lawton pointed out that there appeared to be a lack of standardisation in nurses' assessment and documentation of wounds. Moreover, there was no agreed formal assessment tool recorded in the literature (Lawton 1995). As we discussed in Chapter 3 these difficulties are compounded in the case of intraoral wounds, when not only is physical access limited but the nurse may be even less familiar with what to look for and how to manage particular problems.

## ANATOMY AND PHYSIOLOGY

In this section a knowledge of the basic anatomy and physiology of tissue types will be assumed so that we can devote our thoughts to the dynamics of wound healing, which are essential to the understanding of wound care.

## Healing of incisional wounds

Most commonly these wounds are surgical wounds and the edges are easily approximated. The small amount of blood left in the wound cleft clots and tends to glue the edges together. This process is aided by the normal inflammatory exudation which follows the injury. Within a few hours a single layer of epidermal cells migrates from the skin or mucosal edge to form a delicate covering over the raw area of dermis.

Some 36–72 hours after the wound has been produced the predominant cell in the inflammatory exudate is the macrophage. Macrophage infiltration is followed a day or two later by the proliferation of fibroblasts which produce collagen and other tissue proteins. Also during this period, small capillary buds grow into the wound from intact dermal vessels near the wound edges. This newly vascularised, collagen-producing tissue is called granulation tissue and eventually organises into scar tissue.

## Healing of wounds involving tissue loss

There are few significant differences between the process of wound healing in the incisional wound and those of a tissue defect where the skin edges cannot be approximated, other than those of degree. In this case the wound granulates from the base upwards towards the surface and more scarring results. One feature not seen in relation to incisional wounds is wound contraction.

In open wounds, after 2–3 days the wound area starts to decrease. This is a real movement of the wound margins and is independent of the rate of epithelialisation. The favoured hypothesis is that this contraction is brought about by the action of cells which appear at the wound edges in the first week and which show features of both fibroblasts and smooth muscle cells (myofibroblasts).

## Healing in some specialised tissues

### Bone

The stages of fracture healing are illustrated in Figure 4.1. As with soft tissue there is haematoma formation. The combined presence of blood clot and inflammatory oedema causes some loosening of the periosteal attachment, and a fusiform swelling occurs at the fracture site. After about 4 days the vascular granulation tissue completely replaces the blood clot and extends into the surrounding marrow cavity for a considerable distance

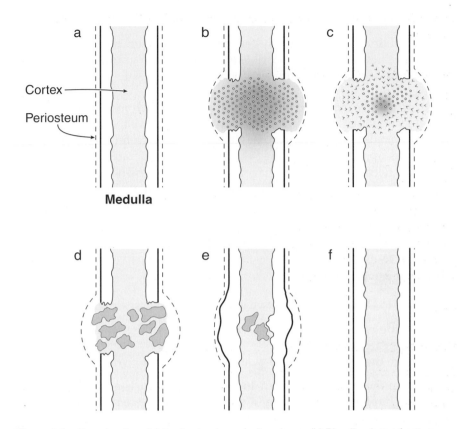

a

Cortex

Periosteum

Medulla

b

c

d

e

f

**Figure 4.1**  Bone healing. (a) Basic structure of a long bone. (b) Bleeding into a fracture. The blood clots, and the periosteum is elevated as a result. There is a brief inflammatory reaction. (c) Granulation tissue is formed. (d) Osteoid and cartilage appear. (e) The callus is replaced by lamellar bone. (f) The new bone is remodelled.

from the fracture line. Within this granulation tissue small groups of cartilage cells form. Subsequently, small islands of cartilage appear, mainly on the periosteal aspect, so that the bone ends are united in a sleeve of granulation tissue and cartilage known as the provisional callus.

At the end of the first week some calcium is deposited in the cartilage islands and osteoblasts begin to form seams of osteoid which traverse the callus. This continues until the callus becomes fully calcified and the bony ends are united by an irregularly shaped bony callus. In the new bone the collagen fibres in the osteoid seams are arranged haphazardly in short bundles, hence the term 'woven bone'. Remodelling of the bone is carried out by osteoclasts. Within 5 weeks an almost new cortex, thicker and as dense as the old, has formed. By 7 weeks the structure of the fractured bone almost completely returns to normal.

*Nervous tissue*

Mitotic activity in the nervous system ceases once neuronal differentiation has been achieved (with the possible exception of the granular layer of the cerebellum). Healing and regeneration of nervous tissue is therefore very limited indeed.

We are mainly interested in peripheral nerves which may be involved in pathology or damaged as the result of surgery to remove the lesion. When an axon is severed it swells and becomes irregular. The myelin sheath splits and later breaks up. The surrounding Schwann cells proliferate and accumulate some lipid released from the damaged myelin. Soon new neurofibrils start to sprout from the proximal end of the axon and invaginate the Schwann cells which act as a guide for the new fibrils. The fibrils push their way down through the Schwann cells at about 1 mm/day. Eventually they may reach the appropriate end organ and some degree of recovery is possible.

## ASSESSMENT

According to Dealey (1994) the two aims of wound assessment are:

• to provide baseline information about the state of the wound so that progress can be monitored
• to ensure that an appropriate wound management product is selected.

How are these aims achieved? In general terms, it is as we have advocated in Chapters 2 and 3 – by a thorough and systematic history and examination of the patient.

## History

In the case of surgical wounds we will have a good idea of the nature of the wound both from the patient's records and from the experience of nursing other patients with similar problems. In the case of traumatic wounds, however, the circumstances under which the injury was sustained may be of great importance to the definitive management. The likelihood of infection from a dog bite, the social implications of interpersonal violence, or the unexplained loss of consciousness in the elderly are all obvious examples in which as much detail as possible needs to be collected from the accident and emergency staff, accompanying persons and the patient him- or herself.

*Medical history*

Again at the risk of being repetitive and stating the obvious, the value of a good medical history cannot be overstated. Diseases such as diabetes mellitus, vascular insufficiency, anaemia, malignancy and immunosuppression all influence the rate of healing. The patient's regular medications and any known allergies may also determine the choice of treatment regimen for a particular wound.

## Visual examination

### Site

Clearly a wound in an area that is subjected to repeated trauma or stretching movements may take longer to heal than one in a flat, immobile part of the body. Furthermore, some areas of the body have a better blood supply than others. Fortunately, the head and neck are well supplied, although it must be remembered that some patients may have had this supply compromised by presurgical radiotherapy.

### Depth

Wounds can be classified according to the structures that are damaged. Superficial wounds involve only the epidermis. Partial thickness wounds penetrate the epidermis and the dermis, exposing nerve endings. Such wounds are moist and painful. A full thickness wound involves the total loss of the epidermis and dermis, extending into subcutaneous tissues and sometimes into muscle, fascia and even bone.

### Colour

A wound classification system based on colour is helpful but needs to be used in conjunction with other methods of assessment such as the Braden Risk Assessment Scale.

**The black wound.** This usually indicates the presence of foreign material or necrotic tissue. It may completely cover a wound or appear in patches. There is an increased risk of infection, and necrotic tissue must be removed before granulation can occur (Plate 7).

**The yellow wound.** This term is usually reserved for a wound that is covered in slough. Slough is a stringy, necrotic tissue which tends to adhere to the wound base or edges. It can be yellow, white-yellow, grey or brown and is an accumulation of dead cellular debris (Plate 8).

**The green wound.** Infected wounds fall into this category, although not all infected wounds are green. Additional signs of infection such as pain, swelling, heat, redness and fever may be present.

**The red wound.** This characterises the healthy granulating wound (Plate 9). When the granulation tissue is level with the skin surface, epithelial migration takes place (Plate 10) and the wound is covered with new skin or mucosa.

# Wound measurement

Wound measurement serves three purposes (Vowden 1995):

- to document progress in an individual wound as part of treatment or assessment
- to assess the efficacy in terms of wound healing of a dressing or drug therapy
- to predict healing time.

The techniques available for wound measurement are listed in Box 4.1. They are as follows.

## Area measurement

**Linear measurement.** The most common method of calculating area is by measuring the length and width of the wound. This can be inaccurate (Majeske 1992), and Dealey (1994) suggests that this only be used for regular-shaped wounds.

**Tracing.** Open wounds can be measured by tracing the perimeter onto an acetate film with or without a grid (Fig. 4.2). Two-layer versions are available: the tracing is made on the upper layer, and the lower layer, which has been in contact with the wound, is discarded. The calculations can then be tedious, and a hand-held planimeter can be more accurate (Majeske 1992). If a digitiser and a computer are employed then the process can be less onerous.

**Photography.** Photography provides a non-contact method of measuring area and healing. Comparable measurements can be obtained by using it in combination with the above methods (Etris et al 1994). Obviously, standardised conditions must be used.

---

**Box 4.1**   Wound measurement techniques

- Contact
     Tracing overlays and contour
     Depth gauges
     Volume: moulding or liquid
- Non-contact
     Photography
     Stereophotogrammetry
     Video-image analysis
     Structured light
     Laser triangulation

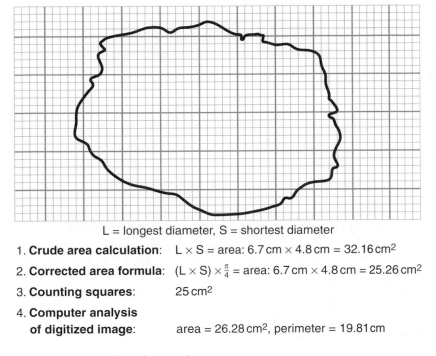

L = longest diameter, S = shortest diameter

1. **Crude area calculation**:   L × S = area: 6.7 cm × 4.8 cm = 32.16 cm$^2$

2. **Corrected area formula**:   (L × S) × $\frac{\pi}{4}$ = area: 6.7 cm × 4.8 cm = 25.26 cm$^2$

3. **Counting squares**:         25 cm$^2$

4. **Computer analysis
   of digitized image**:         area = 26.28 cm$^2$, perimeter = 19.81 cm

**Figure 4.2**   Acetate tracing of a wound.

### Volume measurement

Most wounds are on curved surfaces and therefore require a three dimensional means of assessment. Wound gauges have been used for this purpose (Kundin 1989) but have been shown to consistently underestimate the size of larger wounds (Thomas & Wysocki 1990). To overcome these inaccuracies various methods of filling the wound have been tried. These were reviewed by Plassman (1995), who concluded that, although more accurate than ruler-based techniques, they were still subject to significant error.

Photographic methods can be enhanced to allow measurement of wound volume as well as area. For example, a three dimensional picture can be obtained from two photographs taken simultaneously from different angles. Extra information, such as maximum depth and perimeter, can be obtained from video systems (Smith et al 1992). Furthermore, colour analysis is possible with this system, and some workers consider this to be more important than wound size when evaluating the effects of various treatments (Boardman et al, 1994).

A computer-generated, three dimensional image of a wound can be produced by laser triangulation using a displacement image (Patete & Smith 1994). This method shares the common problems of other non-contact tools: the need to reconstruct the normal skin surface and the inability to deal with undermining.

## PLANNING

The accurate documentation of wounds is now recognised as an essential part of wound management. Unfortunately, research suggests a deficiency in nurses' documentation in this area (Hon & Jones 1996). In the same paper the editors highlight the need to find out why nurses do not document their assessment of wounds as recommended by wound care specialists. Certainly in the head and neck region, where wound assessment and management may be even more difficult than in other parts of the body, we must be willing to work alongside our colleagues in tissue viability and other related disciplines and take their advice as appropriate.

## IMPLEMENTATION

Over the last 40 years the methods of managing wounds have changed dramatically. In particular the routine application of wound dressings has emerged. The more recent concept of moist wound healing has led to the creation of literally hundreds of different cleansing solutions and dressings. Obviously, the specific management of a wound is entirely dependent on the assessment described in the earlier part of this chapter, so we will confine our discussion to some of the more common scenarios encountered in the head and neck unit.

### Wound closure

The methods of wound closure are no different in head and neck surgery than in other areas of surgery, and it would be inappropriate to describe the range of sutures, clips and techniques available. It is worth remembering, however, that from an aesthetic point of view, wounds in this region, particularly on the face, must be neat and every effort made to minimise unattractive scars. Resorbable sutures are generally used for intraoral wounds, and 5/0 or 6/0 monofilament sutures are preferred for the skin of the face.

### Suture removal

Due to the profuse blood supply of the head and neck, wounds tend to heal quickly, and often sutures can be removed from the face on the fifth postoperative day. If the tissues are under more tension, as for example after neck dissections, then they are left for the more conventional 7–10 days and alternate sutures removed if there is any doubt about the strength of the wound closure.

## Wound cleansing

### Technique

To swab or to irrigate? This seems to be the crux of the debate, and as usual there is no absolute answer!

There is a danger with swabbing that granulating and epithelialising tissue may be damaged. Nevertheless, slough and necrotic tissue must be removed to allow healing to take place. The critical factor therefore is the amount of pressure that needs to be applied to achieve the desired result. If the slough/necrotic tissue is very adherent, further soaking, hydrocolloid or hydrogel dressings may be helpful.

The pressure applied when irrigating a wound is also important. For example, the high pressure from a jet of water may well damage healthy granulating tissue. Commercial products such as Steripod® (Seton) and Irricens® (Convatec) have been designed to eliminate the need for supplementary equipment such as syringes and needles, thus minimising the danger of excessive pressures. Needless to say, bleeding wounds are unsuitable for irrigation, and one must always bear in mind the potential discomfort to the patient if nerve endings are likely to be exposed in the wound.

### Cleansing solutions

**Antiseptics.** Antiseptics have an adverse effect on wound healing. They retard both wound contraction and epithelialisation as well as decrease wound tensile strength. The current recommendation in the literature, therefore, is to avoid using antiseptics in open wounds and to use them for what they were originally intended: the disinfection of intact skin (Brown & Zitelli 1995).

**Cetrimide.** Cetrimide has a wide range of bacterial activity. It is often combined with chlorhexidine, and these products are used for their detergent properties, most commonly in the accident and emergency department, for cleaning dirty wounds.

**Chlorinated solutions.** The *British National Formulary* no longer recommends these solutions. They have many disadvantages, and modern alternatives such as hydrogels and hydrocolloids render them obsolete.

**Chlorhexidine.** See Chapter 3.

**Dyes.** Traditionally, dyes were used as astringents to dry macerated skin around wounds and for their antimicrobial properties. Their use is now declining due to lack of data on their clinical effectiveness and fears that they inhibit wound healing. As with the chlorinated solutions they are only mentioned for their historical interest.

**Hydrogen peroxide.** Hydrogen peroxide deserves attention only because it is so commonly used on wounds. Its bacterial potency is minimal at best (Lineweaver et al 1985), and it has been shown to delay wound healing in both animal and human wounds as mentioned in Chapter 3.

**Povidone iodine.** Povidone iodine has the broadest spectrum of any antiseptic commonly available. Its antibacterial effect is reduced by contact with pus and exudate, so preparations must be applied at intervals sufficiently short for the brown coloration to persist. It has a low risk of sensitivity.

**Proflavine.** Proflavine cream has been used to soak gauze to pack wound cavities. In the form of an oil-in-water emulsion it has a mildly bacteriostatic effect. It does not seem to offer any advantage over modern alternatives such as calcium alginate (Gupta et al 1991) or xeroform petrolatum with 3% bismuth tribromophenate, which is commonly used in the USA.

**Silver nitrate.** Silver nitrate has a broad antibacterial spectrum. It is only used occasionally in stick or cream form for the treatment of hypergranulation, but it is caustic and its prolonged use is not recommended.

**Sodium chloride.** A 0.9% saline solution is probably the least harmful cleansing agent. It has no antiseptic properties.

**Varidase.** Varidase is an enzymatic debriding agent. It contains streptokinase and streptodornase, which degrade fibrin found in necrotic material.

**Tap water.** At least one study has suggested that tap water is as effective in wound cleansing as sterile saline (Angeras et al 1992).

### Cleansing equipment

According to the Surgical Materials Testing Laboratory (SMTL 1992), non-woven gauze is the most suitable material for swabbing wounds. Cotton wool has the problem of fibre loss, and the fibres act as a focus for infection. The associated inflammatory response delays wound healing.

The debate on whether to use a gloved hand as opposed to forceps has lacked substance and conclusion. It would seem that as long as standard aseptic techniques are adhered to, the instrumentation is of no consequence.

## The superficial incisional surgical site infection

The management of this problem is well described by the Surgical Wound Infection Taskforce (1994). After careful assessment including probing and sampling for culture and sensitivity, this involves the following.

*Antibiotic therapy*

Systemic antimicrobial therapy is indicated where there is cellulitis to the surrounding tissues. There are a number of proprietary antimicrobial sprays and other topical applications commercially available but there is so much variation in opinion on different regimens and their efficacy that they will not be discussed further here.

*Wound drainage*

If gentle manual pressure to the edges of the wound fails to release any discharge then further observation may be all that is required. On the other hand, however, if large amounts of discharge are present then the insertion of an appropriate drain may be necessary. This allows observation of the discharge and keeps the patient clean and dry. Once drainage has stopped, the resulting cavity can be filled with an alginate dressing and covered with an absorbent secondary dressing.

*Reclosure of the wound*

If the wound is superficially open, the edges can be realigned with a subcuticular suture or skin tapes. If the wound gapes throughout its length when probed then it is likely that the wound will require surgical exploration and management.

## The necrotic and sloughy wound

The appearance of slough and/or necrotic tissue in the wound indicates that there has been a deviation from the normal healing process. This tissue renders the wound more susceptible to infection and delays healing by prolonging the inflammatory process. Moreover, the underlying tissue will continue to die.

The aim of wound management, therefore, is to remove the slough and necrotic tissue whilst causing as little damage as possible to the tissue below. Surgical debridement is a quick and efficient way of removing necrotic tissue, although a general anaesthetic may be required, and will be dependent on the patient's general condition.

Enzyme preparations, hydrocolloids or hydrogels, all of which rehydrate the eschar but do not affect the healthy tissue during the separation, may be applied topically. Scoring the hard eschar with a scalpel prior to these applications also helps. The primary dressing should always be covered with a layer of waterproof material to prevent the dressing drying out and adhering to the wound, causing pain and trauma on removal. In the case of the sloughy wound, which usually produces an excess of exudate, an absorbent dressing is indicated.

## The malodorous wound

For patients and their relatives the effect of living with a foul smelling wound is devastating. The main causative factor in these cases is the presence of slough which predisposes the wound to secondary infection. *Bacteroides* and *Clostridium welchii* are anaerobic organisms that produce distinctive odours, as do the aerobic *Proteus*, *Klebsiella* and *Pseudomonas*.

The most frequently documented malodorous wound is the fungating wound (Grocott 1995). Often wound healing is not achievable and management is based on symptom control. Clearly, effective debridement and cleansing as described earlier may be efficacious in itself, but often antibiotic therapy is necessary. If infection has been identified then appropriate systemic antibiotics are used, although topical preparations such as metronidazole gel are a very useful adjunct (O'Rourke 1991).

If it is not possible to eradicate the odour then odour-absorbing dressings may be of some help. These are usually manufactured as an activated charcoal cloth, examples of which are Actisorb Plus®, Kaltocarb® and Lyofoam C®.

## The cavity wound

Although these are less common now in head and neck surgery because of the increasing use of free flap reconstructive techniques, one still occasionally encounters patients with large intraoral defects, for example postmaxillectomy, which are eventually obturated with a removable prosthesis. In the immediate postoperative period the care of the cavity is of paramount importance since the cavity has been surgically designed to offer maximum retention to the proposed obturator and may contain newly placed titanium implants. The successful osseointegration of the latter is very dependent on the absence of infected and necrotic tissue.

Immediately after surgery these cavities are packed with ribbon gauze soaked in Whitehead's varnish.

## The intraoral tissue flap

Following intraoral flap surgery, patients are kept 'nil by mouth' for several days. There are two reasons for this: firstly, to keep the mouth at rest and thus protect the blood supply to the flap; secondly, the wound edges and suture line need to be kept clean and free of food debris which would predispose to infection. During this period the dental hygienist can assist the patient with oral hygiene, and of course the patient needs to be fed either nasogastrically or via a gastrostomy (see Ch. 5).

## Leech therapy

The medicinal leech *Hirudo medicinalis* is a small invertebrate which feeds by sucking blood from a mammalian host. Use is made of this fact in the management of tissue flaps that are compromised by venous congestion. The care and application of leeches is well described by Peel (1993), and there is at least one case report of their successful use in a life-threatening macroglossia (Smeets & Engelberts 1995).

# EVALUATION

Wound management is a dynamic process. Estimates that it costs the NHS about £950M a year put the need for efficient practice in this area sharply into focus. We can only achieve this level of care if we apply the same vigorous clinical audit that we have advocated in each chapter of this book: starting with accurate assessment tools and using them over and over again, as often as is necessary, until the optimal clinical outcome has been achieved.

Patient cooperation is of course vital and this needs to be integrated with a multidisciplinary approach, coordinated by the nurse. In order to carry out this role, nurses need to communicate in a universal language and provide credible reference tools to be shared with other related professionals. We then need to take advantage of the recent upsurge of interprofessional activity in wound care and be willing participants in joint educational programmes (West & Priestly 1994).

REFERENCES

Angeras M H, Brandberg A, Falk A, Seeman T 1992 Comparison between sterile saline and tap water for the cleaning of acute traumatic soft tissue wounds. European Journal of Surgery 133: 597–600

Boardman M, Melhuish J M, Palmer K, Harding K G 1994 Hue, saturation and intensity in the healing wound image. Journal of Wound Care 3(7): 314–319

Brown C D, Zitelli A 1995 Choice of wound dressings and ointments. Otolaryngologic Clinics of North America 28(5): 1081–1091

Dealey C 1994 The care of wounds. Blackwell Scientific, London, p 65

Etris M B, Pribbles J, LaBrecque J 1994 Evaluation of two wound measurement methods in a multi-center, controlled study. Wounds: A Compendium of Clinical Research and Practice 6(3): 107–111

Grocott P 1995 The palliative management of fungating malignant wounds. Journal of Wound Care 4(5): 240–242

Gupta R, Foster M E, Miller E 1991 Calcium alginate in the management of acute surgical wounds and abscesses. Journal of Tissue Viability 1(4): 115–116

Hon J, Jones C 1996 The documentation of wounds in an acute hospital setting. British Journal of Nursing 5(17): 1040–1045

Kundin J I 1989 A new way to size up a wound. American Journal of Nursing 89: 206–207

Lawton L 1995 Assessment variations. Nursing Times 91(30): 58–64

Lineweaver W, Howard R, Soucy D 1985 Topical antimicrobial toxicity. Archives of Surgery 120: 267

Majeske C 1992 Reliability of wound surface area measurements. Physical Therapy 72(2): 138–141

O'Rourke M E 1991 Eliminating odours associated with necrotic lesions. Oncology Nurse Forum 18(1): 134

Patete P, Smith D 1994 Abstract: A non-invasive 3-dimensional diagnostic sound/laser imaging system for precise analysis of wounds. Wound Repair and Regeneration 2:1, 88

Peel K 1993 Making sense of leeches. Nursing Times 89(27): 34–35

Plassman P 1995 Measuring wounds: a guide to the use of wound measuring techniques. Journal of Wound Care 4(6): 269–272

Smeets I M, Engelberts I 1995 The role of leeches in a case of post-operative life-threatening macroglossia. Journal of Laryngology and Otology 109(5): 442–444

Smith D J, Bhat S, Bulgrin J P 1992 Video image analysis of wound repair. Wounds: A Compendium of Clinical Research and Practice 4(1): 6–15

Surgical Materials Testing Laboratory Leaflet 1992 The dressing times. SMTL 5(2): 3

Surgical Wound Infection Task Force 1994 Understanding surgical site infections. Nursing 24(7): 22

Sutton J 1989 Accurate wound assessment. Nursing Times 85(36): 68–71

Thomas A C, Wysocki A B 1990 The healing wound: a comparison of three clinically useful methods of measurement. Decubitus 3: 18–25

Turner V 1991 Standardisation of wound care. Nursing Standard 5(19): 25–28

Vowden K 1995 Common problems in wound care: wound and ulcer measurement. British Journal of Nursing 4(13): 775–779

West P, Priestly J 1994 Working together. Surgical Nurse 7(2): 29–30

# 5

# Nutritional considerations

'It's a very odd thing
As odd as can be
That whatever Miss T. eats
Turns into Miss T.'

Walter de la Mare

KEY POINTS

- Nutritional status – is it important?
- Swallowing assessment
- Enteral feeding – NG or PEG?

## INTRODUCTION

The ability to eat and drink is not simply a functional process. It is a pleasurable activity usually enjoyed in the company of others, and any significant impairment of it has serious effects on the patient's quality of life. In nursing head and neck patients we see many who have problems with oral feeding. The most common conditions leading to such problems include the following.

**Malignancies of the aerodigestive tract.** Clearly, on the basis of anatomical site, patients with carcinomas involving the mouth or throat will often experience difficulty with swallowing (Fig. 5.1). Certainly after resection of such tumours, even with good reconstructive surgery, feeding problems present a challenge to the head and neck nurse.

**Facial trauma.** Fractures of the mandible and maxilla often result in a malocclusion of the teeth which, along with the attendant soft tissue swelling and muscle spasm, make chewing difficult. Although less common nowadays these fractures can be indirectly fixed with elastic or wire intermaxillary fixation which involves splinting the jaws together for peri-

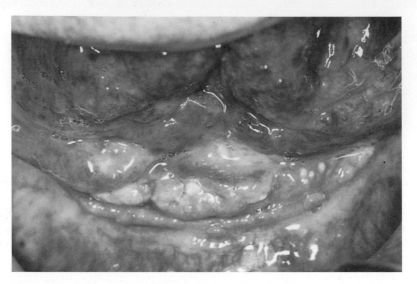

**Figure 5.1**   An intraoral carcinoma in the floor of the mouth.

ods of up to 6 weeks (Fig. 5.2). Malar complex fractures may also interfere with mandibular movement and limit opening thus restricting dietary intake.

**Orthognathic surgery.**  Surgical repositioning of either the upper and/or the lower jaw is now almost routine surgery in many maxillofacial units and, as with trauma patients, intermaxillary fixation may be required and appropriate feeding management undertaken.

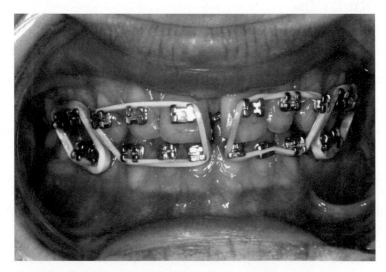

**Figure 5.2**   Intermaxillary fixation.

**Intraoral surgery.** After many intraoral procedures, particularly the placement of free flaps after cancer resections and after cleft palate repairs, it is imperative that the mouth is kept meticulously clean. To that end the patient is often kept 'nil by mouth' for several days after surgery.

**Infective problems.** Patients with peritonsillar abscesses and those with submandibular cellulitis often find it difficult to swallow.

What are the implications of these obstacles to normal feeding? Hussain et al (1996) suggested that individuals who are malnourished on admission to hospital have a protracted stay, experience more complications and are at a greater risk of dying than well nourished individuals with a similar illness. More specifically, individuals with cancer have a relatively high incidence of cachexia. The setting is one in which oral intake of nutrients is insufficient to meet increased energy requirements as a result of a variety of causes. In addition to diminished oral intake, catabolic factors secreted by the tumour – such as cytokine tumour necrosis factor, interleukins, interferon-gamma or cancer cachexia factor 24K (Wilkes 1995, Todorov et al 1996) – head and neck cancer patients are at particular risk from malnutrition for several reasons. Poor dietary habits together with excessive smoking and alcohol consumption are frequently observed. Moreover, the location of the tumour can lead to dysphagia and odynophagia, resulting in a reduced dietary intake. Malnutrition is estimated as occurring in 30–50% of individuals with head and neck malignancies, particularly squamous cell carcinomas of the oropharyngeal and hypopharyngeal area. Furthermore, nutritional depletion has been shown to reduce tolerance to treatment (Bokhorst 1997).

## ANATOMY AND PHYSIOLOGY
## Swallowing

The process of swallowing involves complex neuromuscular coordination of the organs of the upper aerodigestive tract, which all takes place during a brief pause in respiration. The fact that this process takes place thirty-five times an hour whilst awake and six times an hour during sleeping, is a pointer to the significance of interfering with it as of course happens with the resection of head and neck cancer. For descriptive purposes deglutition can be divided into three phases.

### Oral phase

This phase is subdivided into a preparatory phase and a phase which initiates swallowing.

**Preparatory phase.** At this stage the motor control of the tongue is the most important factor. The food is mixed and redistributed from the dependent parts of the mouth to the occlusal surfaces of the teeth. Clearly, intact sensation of the oral buccal mucosa (supplied by cranial nerves V, IX and X) is necessary for efficient manipulation of the bolus. Rotary, lateral and vertical motion of the mandible contributes to the grinding and crushing of food, whilst the maxilla of course remains stationary. Throughout the chewing process the soft palate bulges forwards to prevent premature leakage of the food into the pharynx. The preparatory phase is complete when the food is adequately mixed with saliva and of an appropriate consistency for swallowing.

**Swallowing phase.** This phase begins when a bolus of food is gathered on the dorsal surface of the tongue and lasts for about one second. The tip of the tongue contacts the anterior part of the hard palate, the lateral borders of the tongue curve upwards, and the posterior tongue forms a seal with the soft palate and faucial pillars. The bolus, thus enclosed, is then pushed backwards by a rolling motion of the tongue on the palate from front to back. Although this phase is automatic it is largely under the voluntary control of cranial nerves V, VII and XII.

### Pharyngeal phase

This phase is the start of the involuntary component of swallowing. The initiating mechanism is unclear but is thought to involve IX and X relaying messages to the reticular substance of the upper medulla (Logemann 1988). The four key components of the pharyngeal phase are:

1. closure of the nasopharynx by the approximation of the soft palate to the posterior pharyngeal wall
2. elevation and closure of the larynx
3. contraction of the pharyngeal constrictors
4. opening of the cricopharyngeal muscle (upper oesophageal sphincter).

Laryngeal closure occurs only at the level of the epiglottis. It begins at the true vocal cords and continues upwards to the false cords, the epiglottis and the aryepiglottic folds. This produces a multilayered barrier against aspiration in normal individuals. The larynx moves anteriorly and superiorly to a position under the tongue. The tongue base then moves backward, forcing the bolus onwards. A peristaltic wave then begins with contraction of the superior constrictor and travels inferiorly to the hypopharynx.

Laryngeal elevation is largely responsible for opening of the cricopharyngeus muscle. This widening of the sphincter creates a negative pressure that combines with the positive tongue pressure to move the bolus into the oesophagus. The total duration of pharyngeal activity is about one second.

### Oesophageal phase

This stage of swallow is characterised by a peristaltic wave that travels the length of the oesophagus at about 3–4 cm/s to carry the bolus to the stomach. The lower oesophageal sphincter (a physiological sphincter) relaxes ahead of the wave. At any given time only one peristaltic wave can exist in the oesophagus. Secondary peristaltic waves occur spontaneously several times an hour and help to clear residue and any refluxed gastric material. Oesophageal transit times increase with age (Logemann 1988).

Surgical resections for cancer of the head and neck result in predictable patterns of dysphagia and aspiration. In addition following trauma or severe surgical stress the metabolic and endocrine response is different (Poulin 1991). The increased production of hormones such as glucagon, insulin, cortisol, catecholamines, vasopressin and aldosterone results in a profound change in protein and energy metabolism (Streat & Hill 1987).

## ASSESSMENT

Broadly speaking the assessment of nutritional problems in head and neck patients has two components. There is a need to assess the patient's nutritional status and to assess the functional problem which is causing the nutritional deficit, which more often than not is a swallowing problem. Other causes include the effects of actual and potential alterations in nutrition that may be related to symptoms (e.g. nausea and vomiting), disease process (e.g. obstruction), treatment and alteration in fluid and electrolyte balance.

## Assessment of nutritional status

The assessment of nutritional status is a complicated process and thankfully usually carried out by the dietician! It is helpful, nevertheless, to have a basic knowledge of the problems involved, the main one of which is that there is no single absolute measure of nutritional status. Furthermore, the parameters used are not very reliable. In fact, malnutrition in head and neck cancer patients can vary between 20% and 67%, depending on the parameter used (van Bokhorst-de van der Schueren et al 1997). Any assessment therefore tends to be a composite of a number of parameters which give a rough picture of the true state of affairs. Some of the means of assessment are mentioned below, but more specialised dietetics sources will give more details for those wanting to take the subject further.

### History and examination

It is often difficult, if at all possible, to get an accurate history from patients about their dietary habits. Most of us are not particularly cognisant of the balance of our diet or the amount we eat on a day-to-day basis and may have some trouble relating it accurately to a nurse. Many of our patients come from disadvantaged social backgrounds and may be even less able to communicate this information or may even be embarrassed to do so. Nevertheless, it is worth taking the time to gather as much information as possible about the patient's usual diet, preferences and eating ability either directly or from accompanying friends and relatives.

As with many other clinical conditions the malnourished patient may present anywhere along a spectrum of clinical features. It almost goes without saying that children stop growing and adults lose weight. The face at first looks younger but later appears old, withered and expressionless. The skin is lax, pale and dry. Hair becomes thin or lost except in adolescents. Subcutaneous fat disappears, skin turgor is lost and muscles waste. The arm circumference is reduced. The patient becomes sensitive to the cold. Psychologically, the individual loses initiative and is often apathetic and depressed.

Undernourished patients are more susceptible to infections, and, with respiratory muscles wasting, there is an increased risk of bronchopneumonia.

The disadvantages of physical examination as a routine method of detecting abnormalities are:

- physical examinations are time-consuming and costly
- data obtained cannot stand alone, therefore further investigation is required
- examiners vary in ability to observe and correctly interpret signs and symptoms
- deficiencies must be severe and/or persistent enough to produce visible symptoms (Bergstrom 1992).

### Anthropometry

Anthropometry, the measurement of the human body, is an additional method of clinical assessment. Anthropometric measurements, such as height, wrist circumference, elbow breadth, weight, triceps, skinfold thickness, upper arm circumference are non-specific indicators of growth and development and nutritional status.

**Height and weight.** Usual and actual body weight (UBW and ABW) are used to calculate percentage weight loss.

*Percentage weight loss (PWL)*

$$PWL = \frac{UBW - ABW}{UBW} \times 100$$

More than 10% weight loss in the last 6 months can be regarded as severe malnutrition (Gottschlich et al 1993).

*Percentage ideal body weight (PIW).* Frame size can be estimated from height and wrist circumference. The PIW can then be computed as the midpoint of the weight range for a given height and frame size from published life insurance tables.

### Serum albumin concentrations

Serum albumin (Alb) is a serological test used for identifying visceral protein depletion. Serum albumin may react within 12–24 hours in an acute catabolic state with poor reserves. Unfortunately, albumin has a long half life (20 days), so a fall in serum albumin is indicative of prolonged severe protein deficiency (Dudack 1993). Serum albumin levels less than 21 g/L are considered to represent severe depletion (Gottschlich et al 1993).

### Total lymphocyte counts

Malnutrition adversely affects immune function, and tests of immune function can assist in determining the extent of malnutrition. These tests involve total lymphocyte count (TLC) and antigen skin tests. However, neither of these tests is commonly used in evaluating individuals, as many variables obscure the findings (Wilkes 1995).

$$\text{TLC} = \frac{\% \text{ lymphocytes} \times \text{white blood cell count}}{100}$$

### Nutritional index

Nutritional index (NI), if used for a group of patients, can be used for comparative studies, with previous studies used as a reference (de Jong et al 1985, von Meyenfeldt et al 1992).

$$\text{NI} = (0.14 \times \text{Albumin (g/L)}) + (0.03 \times \text{PIW (\%)}) + (0.73 \times \text{TLC } (10^9/\text{mm}^3)) - 8.90$$

### Body fat and lean body mass

Estimates of these parameters can be made from measurements of resistance and reactance using bioelectrical impedance analysis (BIA, RJL Systems Inc, Clinton Twp, MI).

## Assessment of swallowing

In addition to the assessment of the degree of malnutrition, it is of equal importance to assess the functional aspect of swallowing. The severity of the swallowing dysfunction can be related to the extent of lingual resection, mobility of residual tongue, type of reconstruction, involvement of other structures, individual motivation and ability to adapt, and the skill of the rehabilitation team. When more than one phase of swallowing is involved the severity of the problem increases.

Initial swallowing assessment includes:

- observation of how the individual patient handles his or her own secretions
- examination of the anatomy, function and sensory response of the oral and pharyngeal structures
- checking for cough, gag and swallow reflexes
- observation for any signs of aspiration
- testing the ability to swallow very small amounts of water and pureed foods (five consecutive swallows, 5–15 mL each).

*Videofluoroscopy*

When swallowing function is disturbed, a videofluoroscope modified barium swallow (Fig. 5.3) should be done and interpreted by the appropriate members of the rehabilitation team (Logemann 1989). The modified barium swallow will provide information about the oral preparatory and oral swallow stages and the pharyngeal stage.

## PLANNING

Planning appropriately in order to meet individual nutritional needs will involve discussion with the patient, the dietician, nursing and medical personnel. In order to prevent the loss of muscle and fat stores it is important to develop and implement an appropriate nutritional plan based on the assessment. The goals of intervention are to restore and maintain protein stores within the body (Wilkes 1995). Maintenance diets are designed to preserve lean body mass and should contain approximately 8% of total calories as protein with a nitrogen ratio of 1:300 (Blackburn & Bristran 1977). Alternatively, anabolic diets replenish lean body mass in malnutrition, stress or disease. In the absence of renal or hepatic disease, maximum protein utilisation is obtained if 16% of the calorie requirement is provided as protein.

In order to achieve appropriate nutritional support, protein, carbohydrates, fats, water, minerals and vitamins must be provided. The optimal amount and balance of components in the individual diet, however, is dependent on the specific goal of the nutritional therapy, the individual's physical status, nutritional assessment results and any attendant pathological processes (Mundy & Panje 1982).

Minimal daily calorific requirements may be roughly estimated using 35 kcal/kg/day for maintenance diets and 45 kcal/kg/day for anabolic diets. The average adult male requires 1800 cal/day. The calorific reserve is derived from muscle and hepatic glycogen (900 cal/day maximum) (Cahill

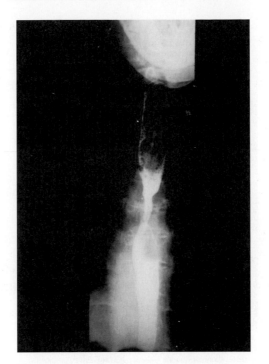

**Figure 5.3**   Radiograph of a barium swallow investigation showing constriction of the oesophagus.

1970). Although it is not always possible to predict which patients will have feeding problems, there are some cases in which there will be no doubt. For example, it is obvious that patients with large oral cancers will have swallowing problems after resection. Clearly, therefore, it is important for the head and neck nurse to have a broad appreciation of some of the surgical procedures which are undertaken. There are some excellent texts which deal with this very subject, but for the sake of completeness some of the commoner procedures are outlined below.

## Common surgical procedures

### Glossectomy

Swallowing problems resulting from glossectomy (Fig. 5.4) depend on the site of resection and the type of reconstruction carried out. The floor of the mouth is often involved, and reconstruction needs to be adapted accordingly. Nowadays, unless the tissue deficit is very small and well defined, repair with microvascular free flap is the treatment of choice. These flaps, however, are adynamic and insensate and tend to create a non-functional

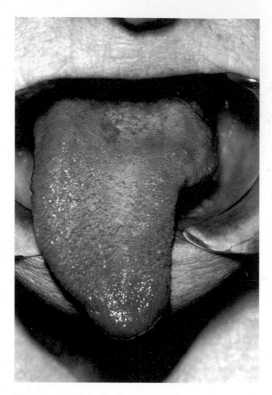

**Figure 5.4**   Tongue after partial glossectomy.

area of dead space in the oral cavity. The use of remaining tongue in the closure of oral defects further reduces the amount of functional tongue and increases masticatory and swallowing difficulties. Ruhl (1997) highlights that, following total glossectomy, diet was restricted and many individuals relied on gastrostomy tubes for nutrition.

### Mandibulectomy

One of the commonest operations carried out in head and neck surgery is the composite resection. In this procedure glossectomy, mandibulectomy and radical neck dissection are carried out for *en bloc* removal of intraoral cancer. In addition to the difficulties created by the glossectomy alone, these patients often experience such swallowing problems postoperatively that drooling is a significant complaint, particularly if the anterior mandible is involved. Additionally, the myohyoid, genioglossus and the suprahyoid musculature are often disrupted. A further contributing factor to postoperative drooling results from the sectioning of the inferior alveolar ridge, labial alveolar mucosa and gingiva, skin and mucous membrane of the lower lip as well as the skin of the chin. The predictable functional reconstruction of the mandible and adjacent soft tissues after oncological surgery has been a difficult problem to solve. However, it is well accepted that the best results are achieved when the deficit is reconstructed primarily. Delayed reconstruction often has limited functional results because of the soft tissue contracture, fibrosis or atrophy of remaining masticatory muscles (Navarro-Vila et al 1996). Additionally, pedicled pectoralis major mycutaneous flaps (PMMF), because of bulkiness and lack of sensation, interfere with postoperative oral function. Soft tissue free flaps (FF) are typically thin, pliable, potentially sensate and at times may even lubricate (Tsue et al, 1997).

## Surgery of the palate

Resection of the hard and/or soft palate is often undertaken for squamous cell and salivary gland malignancies. Tumours of the retromolar regions as well as those of the sinuses or orbits may also require parts of the palate to be included in the resection to ensure clear margins. The resulting defects tend to cause abnormalities in the oral phase of swallowing, and escape of food into the nose may be an additional problem.

Fortunately, the rigid nature of the palate lends itself well to prosthetic obturation, and the prognosis for rehabilitation of swallowing is good. In the case of the soft palate the outlook is less favourable. Although this organ has great ability to adapt to structural changes with time and intensive speech therapy, greater degrees of tissue loss result in dysphagia. Furthermore, palatopharyngeal valve dysfunction occurs in patients following resections that have included the posterior portion of the maxilla. The dysfunction is attributed to destruction of the attachment for, or denervation of, the palatal muscles or the relative shrinkage or immobilisation of the soft palate through scar contracture. Such individuals have poor oronasal separation even when their palatal prosthesis has good stability (Matsui et al 1995).

## Total laryngectomy

Estimates of dysphagia after total laryngectomy range from 10% to 58% (Balfe et al 1982, Nayar et al 1984). Resection includes all laryngeal structures which involves the cricoid and thyroid cartilages, true and false cords, the epiglottis and hyoid bone. A portion of the tongue base is included if the tumour has breached the supraglottic area and extended to the vallecula. Postoperative dysphagia occurs as a result of changes that occur in areas of the pharynx and tongue base – specifically, stenosis in the pharyngo-oesophageal segment and/or physiological alterations in muscle function in this area, giving rise to spasm (Crary & Growasky 1996).

*Partial laryngectomy*

This operation is indicated if the carcinoma is confined to the supraglottic region. It has the advantage of voice preservation and the avoidance of a permanent tracheal stoma. Postoperatively, however, the patient must learn to swallow without aspiration. A temporary tracheostomy is placed at the time of surgery, as is a nasogastric feeding tube. These are removed approximately 10–14 days later, and swallowing studies are generally delayed until this time as the feeding tube is uncomfortable and does not allow full closure of the soft palate against the posterior nasopharyngeal wall.

*Reconstruction of pharynx and cervical oesophagus*

When large amounts of pharyngeal tissue are removed with total laryngectomy, reconstruction is commonly undertaken with a jejunal free flap, gastric pull-up, regional mycutaneous flap, colon interposition or radial forearm flap. Swallowing results with either gastric pull-up or jejunal interposition are superior to those with mycutaneous flap.

The radial forearm free flap spares an intra-abdominal procedure, but swallowing results are not yet well evaluated, and there appears to be a higher rate of stricture and fistula formation (Carlson et al 1993).

*Orthognathic surgery*

Many oral and maxillofacial operations compromise the individual's ability to eat and drink in the early postoperative period. This period varies with the nature and extent of the procedure. Individuals who undergo orthognathic surgery or who have fractured their jaw are unable to take normal diet for 6–8 weeks. Despite dietary advice and support, many continue to lose weight during this period of time, while their jaws are immobilised by intermaxillary fixation and they remain on a soft diet.

*Radiotherapy*

The side effects of radiotherapy such as mucositis and pain have been shown to prevent the individual from being able to eat or drink effectively (McDonough et al 1996). The observed swallowing disorders appear to be due to sluggish contraction of the affected muscles, which make timing uncoordinated and in some cases movement incomplete.

# IMPLEMENTATION

Having formulated a highly individualised plan for feeding the patient with feeding problems what do we do about it? It seems obvious that if the patient can manage to take food orally then that should be the first choice of feeding method. Other methods of enteral feeding are often required if the patient is unable to eat and drink, and of course they can be used to supplement oral intake. If all else fails, the patient can be fed parenterally. The different feeding methods will be discussed below.

## Oral feeding

The oral route is the preferred method of feeding for many reasons, not least for the social, psychological, clinical and economic advantages. Unfortunately a very simplistic approach has often been taken and it has been assumed that the answer to swallowing difficulties was a liquidised diet. No account would be taken of factors such as taste and texture. There is no harm in remembering a few basic hints that have already been adopted into routine practice in most centres.

- Easy to chew does not mean easy to swallow.
- Liquids are usually more difficult to swallow than solids since they do not provide as strong a stimulus. Additionally, water is usually the most difficult to handle, since taste and texture are not stimulated.
- Liquids such as gravy and juices can be used to moisten food. However, because of the nature of dysphagia, liquids and solids may need to be presented separately.

Commonly, however, even with well-motivated patients and staff, it is not possible to maintain adequate nutrition with the standard hospital diet, and supplemental feeding is indicated. This can be done by adding supplements to meals and/or by arranging snacks between meals. Nevertheless, above a certain level of daytime supplementation (which is individual for each patient), appetite and therefore oral food intake is suppressed (Taylor & Goodinson-Mclaren 1992). It is therefore important when evaluating the optimal oral supplement to select one that provides the highest number of calories in the smallest volume (calorie dense). In addition the supplement should have a high protein, carbohydrate and fat content, the latter ideally from medium chain triglycerides.

As well as optimising the content of the patient's oral diet the head and neck team can help with its delivery. Since dysphagia may be due to anatomical alterations following surgery, compensatory methods may need to be implemented in an attempt to improve swallowing. These are described by Casper & Colton (1993) and include:

- tilting the head backward when there is limited anterior–posterior tongue movement; this is helpful in moving the bolus to the back of the mouth
- tilting the head to the more 'normal' side (postsurgical), taking advantage of its more normal function when the impairment is unilateral

- tilting the head forward, which is beneficial for individuals who exhibit delayed swallow reflex, thereby resricting inadvertent passage of the substance into the pharynx valleculae and airway.

### Intraoral exercises

When less than 50% of the tongue has been excised, exercises should be devised to encourage tongue to palate contact. When more than 50% of the tongue has been resected, or mobility is minimal, tongue exercises will be of little value and should not be done until an intraoral prosthesis has been fitted. Jaw- and mouth-opening exercises will be important, however, particularly when radiotherapy is planned.

### Thermal stimulation

When pharyngeal involvement delays triggering of the swallow reflex, thermal stimulation of the anterior faucial pillars may be of benefit.

### Supraglottic swallow technique

This may be beneficial when the larynx is involved either through lack of laryngeal elevation or lack of glottic closure. The individual is taught to hold his or her breath then swallow and release with a sharp cough immediately after the swallow.

## Enteral feeding

When the gastrointestinal tract is functioning and accessible, enteral feeding is a useful means of substituting for or supporting the oral diet. There are numerous methods of administering enteral feeds, including nasogastric, nasoduodenal, nasojejunal, oesophagotomy, pharyngostomy, gastrostomy, jejunostomy and, in individuals following total laryngectomy, a primary tracheo-oesophageal puncture via a tube placed as a stent for maintenance of a fistula. Within this chapter we will deal only with the most common methods of enteral feeding.

### Nasogastric feeding

Nasogastric (NG) feeding tends to be the most common form of tube feeding because it is involuntary and delivers food directly into the stomach. It overcomes most causes of malnutrition resulting from inadequacies in food ingestion. It must be remembered, however, that the primary initial complication of NG intubation is tube misplacement in the respiratory tract, which can lead to life-threatening perforation of the lung or pneumonitis from aspiration.

The introduction of fine bore catheters has reduced some of the mechanical complications of earlier tubes. Prolonged nasal intubation, however, may lead to nasopharyngeal discomfort, and/or mucosal erosion. There is also a potential for increased upper airway resistance and interference with breathing (Taylor & Goodinson-Mclaren 1992). Additionally, accidental displacement of the catheter by the patient and discomfort during replacement of the tube may occur. Furthermore, the position of the tube needs to be checked radiographically each time it is replaced as well as by aspiration of gastric contents prior to each administration of feed. There are also social and psychological implications because of the patient's changed body image.

### Gastrostomy feeding

Feeding tubes can be placed directly into the stomach across the abdominal wall. Most often nowadays this is done endoscopically (percutaneous endoscopic gastrostomy or PEG feeding) – see Figure 5.5. PEG feeding has been used as a postoperative measure when problems with NG feeding have occurred. NG tubes are often poorly tolerated and extubation is common.

PEG under local anaesthetic was first described in 1980 for obtaining access to the stomach in patients requiring long-term feeding (Gauderer et al 1980). Since then, minor modifications of both technique and gastrostomy tubes have allowed PEG to evolve into a standard procedure that is performed in most general hospitals. PEG feeding is well tolerated by patients and has a low morbidity (6–16%) and mortality (0–1%) (Larson et al 1987). There are two main techniques used for the placement of PEG tubes: the 'pull' and 'push' techniques.

**The 'pull' technique** (Fig. 5.6).   After passage of an endoscope, the stomach is insufflated to allow juxtaposition of the anterior abdominal wall. An introducer catheter is then passed through the abdominal wall into the gastric lumen. Visualisation by transillumination from the endoscope light helps determine the appropriate position of the PEG tube. After the introducer catheter is advanced into the gastric lumen it is grasped with an endoscopic snare. A loop guidewire is then introduced and the snare is gently loosened off the catheter and then retightened around the guidewire. The endoscope, the snare and the guidewire are then withdrawn through the mouth, and the tapered end of the PEG tube is attached to the guide wire. The guide wire exiting the abdominal wall is then pulled and the PEG tube exteriorised, leaving the mushroom tip in the gastric lumen, approximating the stomach to the abdominal wall. A bumper or T-bar is then placed at skin level, and the gastroscope is reinserted to verify intragastric position and confirm absence of bleeding or tension at the PEG site.

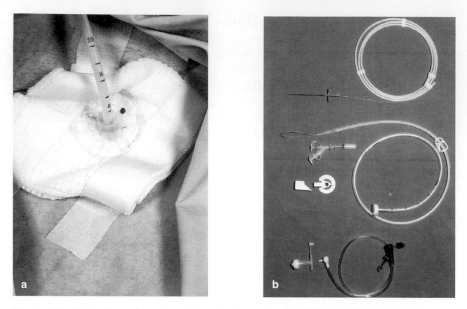

**Figure 5.5**   Percutaneous endoscopic gastrostomy feeding. (a) Area of insertion of tube. (b) Range of tubes and related equipment.

**The 'push' technique** (Fig. 5.7).   This is a modification of the original technique, which uses a guide wire and a stiff dilator which allows the tube to be pushed through the abdominal wall over the guide wire. The guide wire is placed in the same manner as with the pull technique, but the endoscope is removed prior to the placement of the tube.

**Open gastrostomy.** Open gastrostomy would only be considered for patients who were not candidates for or who had failed endoscopic methods. The procedure is so infrequently encountered in head and neck nursing that it will not be discussed any further in this text.

### Tube feeding administration methods

After the most appropriate access route and infusion site have been decided, formula administration can then be considered. Bolus, intermittent or continuous feeding can be delivered when the tube is in the stomach. Bolus or intermittent are more frequently delivered to home care patients to allow them to return to the activities of daily living without being connected to infusion pumps. For hospitalised patients, continuous feedings are the usual method of choice but are not mandatory, depending on the patient's clinical condition and tolerance. The dietician should be involved as early as possible in the overall nutritional management of these patients.

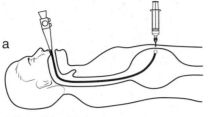
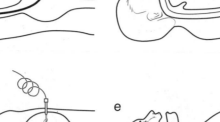
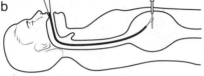
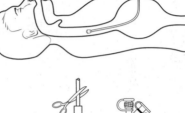
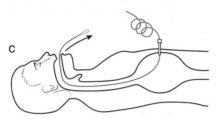
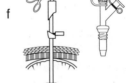
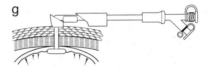

**Figure 5.6**   The 'pull' technique.
(a)  Transillumination of abdominal wall by gastroscope light, and injection of local anaesthetic.
(b)  Cannula and trochar inserted through abdominal wall into stomach, then trochar removed. Guide wire fed through cannula into stomach and grasped by biopsy forceps.
(c)  Gastroscope withdrawn bringing guide wire with it.
(d)  Wire loop on tip of gastrostomy tube attached to the loop of the guide wire.
(e)  Guide wire withdrawn back through the abdominal wall, bringing gastrostomy tube with it.
(f)  Fixation base and cover positioned on tube. Gastrostomy tube cut to convenient length. Corlock-Corport Y-adapter inserted into tube to prevent deflation of retaining balloon.
(g)  Gentle traction exerted on gastrostomy tube, followed by positioning of external fixation device against the abdominal wall.
Source: Corpak Medsystems, Wheeling, Illinois, USA. Redrawn with permission.

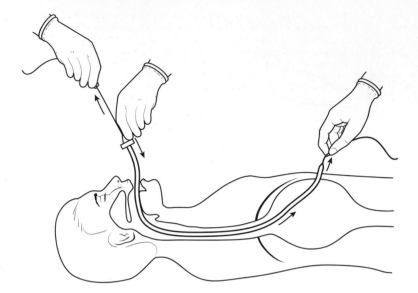

**Figure 5.7** The 'push' technique.

## EVALUATION

In some respects, ongoing evaluation of nutritional management is relatively easy whilst the patient is in hospital. Input and output can be closely monitored and the level of patient compliance with feeding regimens assessed. There is often access to specialist dietetic advice, and much of the data is quantitative and can be analysed on custom-designed software packages. Unfortunately, once the patient goes home the task becomes almost impossible. As we have discussed, many patients, particularly those with oral malignancy, are not from optimal social backgrounds and many return to their old aetiological habits. Furthermore, these patients are, by definition, in the older age groups and may not have a high level of family support for tasks such as changing and maintaining feeding tubes.

Notwithstanding these difficulties, it is our responsibility to 'close the audit loop' as far as possible. It is likely that the best way forward in this connection is to offer as much support as possible to the development of a multidisciplinary approach to nutritional management and to develop ever-closer links with the primary care team so that the patient is managed on the same principles at both the inpatient and outpatient stages.

REFERENCES

Balfe D M, Koehler R E, Setzen M, Weyman P J, Baron R L, Ogura J H 1982 Barium examination of the oesophagus after total laryngectomy. Radiology 143: 501–508

Bergstrom N 1992 Measuring dietary intake and nutritional outcomes. In: Frank-Stromberg (ed) Instruments for clinical nursing research. Jones Bartlett, London, ch 14

Blackburn G L, Bristran B R 1977 Curative nutrition: protein calorie management. In: Nutritional support of medical practice. Harper & Row, London

Bokhorst M A E 1997 Assessment of malnutrition in head and neck cancer and their relation to post operative complications. Head and Neck 19(5): 419–425

Cahill G F 1970 Starvation in man. New England Journal of Medicine 282(12): 668–675

Carlson G W, Coleman J J, Jurkiewicz M J 1993 Reconstruction of the hypopharynx and cervical oesophagus. Current Problems in Surgery 30(5): 425–480

Casper J K, Colton R H 1993 Clinical manual for laryngectomy and head and neck cancer rehabilitation. Singular, California

Crary M A, Growasky A L 1996 Using botulinium toxin a to improve speech and swallowing function following total laryngectomy. Archives of Otolaryngology–Head and Neck Surgery 122(7): 760–763

de Jong P C M, Wesdrop R I C, Volovics A, Rouflart M, Greep J M, Soeters P B 1985 The value of objective measurements to select patients who are malnourished. Clinical Nutrition 4: 61–66

Dudack S G 1993 Nutrition handbook for nursing practice, 2nd edn. J B Lippincott, Philadelphia

Gauderer M W L, Ponsky I L, Izant R J 1980 Gastrostomy with laparotomy: a percutaneous endoscopic technique for feeding gastrostomy. Journal of Pediatric Surgery 15: 872–875

Gottschlich M M, Matarese L E, Shronto E P 1993 Nutrition support dietetics core curriculum, 2nd edn. American Society for Parenteral and Enteral Nutrition, Silver Spring, MD

Hussain A Wolfcey S, Massey J, Geddes A, Cox J 1996 Percutaneous endoscopic gastrostomy. Postgraduate Medical Journal 76: 581–585

Larson D E, Burton D D, Schroeder K W et al 1987 Percutaneous endoscopic gastrostomy. Gastroenterology 93: 48–52

Logemann J A 1988 Swallowing physiology and pathophysiology. Otolaryngological Clinics of North America 21(4): 613–623

Logemann J A 1989 Speech and swallowing rehabilitation for head and neck tumour patients. In: Myers E N S, Suen J Y (eds) Cancer of the head and neck, 2nd edn. Churchill Livingstone, New York, pp 1021–1043

Matsui K, Ohno K, Shirota T, Imai S, Yanashita Y, Michi K 1995 Speech function following maxillectomy reconstructed by rectus mycutaneous flap. Journal of Cranio-Maxillo-Facial Surgery 23(3): 160–164

McDonough E M, Varvares M A, Dunphy F R, Dunleary T R N, Dunphig C H, Boyd J H 1996 Changes in quality of life scores in a population of patients treated for squamous cell carcinoma of the head and neck. Head and Neck 18(6): 487–493

Mundy J C, Panje W R 1982 Nutrition in head and neck surgery. American Journal of Otolaryngology 3: 41–47

Navarro-Vila C, Bonja-Morant A, Cuesta M, Lopez de Atalya F J, Ignacio Salmeron J, Barrios M 1996 Aesthetic and function reconstruction with the trapezius osseomycutaneous flap and dental implants in oral cavity cancer patients. Journal of Cranio-Maxillo-Facial Surgery 24(6): 322–329

Nayar R C, Sharma V P, Aora M M L 1984 A study of the pharynx after laryngectomy. Journal of Laryngology and Otology 98: 807–810

Poulin E 1991 Prophylactic nutrition. Canadian Journal of Surgery 34: 555

Ruhl C M 1997 Survival function and quality of life after total glossectomy. The Laryngoscope 107(10): 1316–1321

Streat S J, Hill G L 1987 Nutritional support in the management of critically ill patients in surgical intensive care. World Journal of Surgery 11: 194

Taylor S, Goodinson-Mclaren S 1992 Nutritional support: a team approach. Wolfe, London

Todorov P, Cariuk P, McDevitt T, Coles B, Fearon K, Fisdale M 1996 Characterisation of a cancer cachetic factor. Nature 379: 739–742

Tsue T T, Desyatnikora S S, Deleyiannis F W, Futran N D, Stack B C, Weymuller E A Jr, Glenn M G 1997 Comparison of cost and function in reconstruction of posterior oral cavity and oropharynx. Archives of Otolaryngology–Head and Neck Surgery 123(7): 731–737 van Bokhorst-de van der Schueren M A, van Leeuwen P A, Sauerwein H P, Kuik D J, Snow G B, Quak J J 1997 Assessment of malnutrition parameters in head and neck cancer and their relation to post operative complications. Head and Neck 19(5): 419–425

von Meyenfeldt M F, Meijerink W J H J, Rouflart M M J, Buil-Maasen M T H J, Soeters P B 1992 Perioperative nutritional support: a randomised clinical trial. Clinical Nutrition 1: 180–186

Wilkes G M 1995 Cancer and HIV clinical nutrition pocket guide. Jones and Bartlett, London

# 6

# Acute postoperative pain

'It would be a great thing to understand pain in all its meanings'
Peter Mere Lathan

---

KEY POINTS

- Head and neck pain – the nursing challenge
- Pain measurement tools
- Methods of pain control
- Specific head and neck pain studies
- Acute pain services

---

## INTRODUCTION

Alleviation of pain is an important aspect of nursing care, and a great deal of attention has been paid to it in recent professional literature. It is disappointing, however, to have the clinical impression confirmed by several authors that many patients in the latter part of the 20th century continue to experience considerable postoperative pain and discomfort (Commission on the Provision of Surgical Services 1990, Kuhn et al 1990). This severe indictment must act as a spur to improve this area of patient care. Effective methods of pain control are available and widely advocated but, sadly, are often not implemented. With the changing face of surgical practice and more cases being carried out on a day-care or outpatient basis, it is now even more important that analgesia is well managed.

The implications of poorly controlled postoperative pain are significant. The resultant adverse effects include pulmonary, cardiovascular, gastrointestinal and urinary dysfunction, impairment of muscle metabolism and function, as well as neuroendocrine and metabolic changes (Ready 1994). Furthermore, postoperative pain is a source of fear and anxiety in hospitalised patients (Caunt 1992) and can lead to anger and resentment if prolonged. The pain experience may be exacerbated, and insomnia can result, with further detriment to recovery. Clearly, this is of particular importance in patients who have undergone major head and neck procedures where self-image is distorted and the ability to communicate verbally is often impaired.

Another consideration for head and neck surgical patients is that they may well have had simultaneous surgery on other regions, for example the harvesting of skin, rib, or iliac crest bone.

Why do we still have problems managing postoperative pain? There are a number of contributing factors, but the most obvious is poor communication and feedback between members of staff and with the patient. Although doctors prescribe analgesia it is the nurses' role to administer it and ensure patient comfort. It is usually the nurse who assesses the patient's pain and makes the decision as to whether to administer 'prn' analgesia and when. His or her attitude towards pain is therefore very significant indeed. There are misconceptions held by many nurses of the risks of dependence and respiratory depression associated with the use of post-operative analgesia. A study carried out by Mackintosh (1994) showed alarming gaps in the knowledge of ITU and hospice nursing staff of pain control methods and efficacy of commonly used analgesics. Other workers have shown that the nurse's attitude to pain may influence the patient's needs (Davitz & Pendleton 1969).

## ANATOMY AND PHYSIOLOGY

The International Association for the Study of Pain has defined pain as 'an unpleasant sensory and emotional experience with actual or potential tissue damage, or described in terms of such damage' (Merskey et al 1979).

Surgery produces local tissue damage with consequent release of algesic substances, including prostaglandins, histamine, serotonin, bradykinin and substance P. These generate noxious stimuli that are transduced by nociceptors and transmitted by two fibre systems to the central nervous system, where they are modulated according to the Gate theory.

The A-delta fibres are small, myelinated fibres which transmit at twice the rate of the finer, unmyelinated C-fibres, and transmit sharp, well-localised painful stimuli. The C-fibres relay dull, aching and diffuse stimuli. Further transmission is determined by complex modulating influences in the spinal cord and the brain.

Of particular interest to the head and neck team is the trigeminal or fifth cranial nerve. This is the major somatic sensory nerve of the face, the anterior half of the scalp, the mouth cavity, the meninges, the sinuses, the tongue, the cornea and the outer surface of the eardrum. It transmits the sensations of pain and temperature and all kinds of touch, pressure and proprioception along the pathways that are shown in Figure 6.1. General

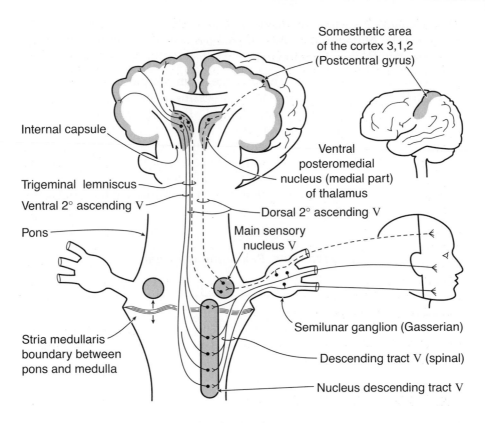

**Figure 6.1**    Pain pathways from the head and neck.

sensations from small areas of the back of the ear and external auditory meatus are supplied by components of cranial nerves VII (facial), IX (glossopharyngeal) and X (vagus). The axons of these nerves enter the (descending) spinal tract of the Vth nerve and then follow the same pathway as the trigeminal fibres.

## ASSESSMENT

The clinical assessment of pain from a qualitative point of view is often not difficult. The signs are well recognised:

- pallor
- sweating
- tachycardia
- elevated blood pressure
- behavioural changes such as moaning, crying, restlessness
- changes in facial expression.

The quantitative measurement of pain is, however, much more of a problem. The literature identifies three major types of measurement used to assess pain. These are summarised by Kitson (1994) as follows.

• *Pain measurement tools.* These range from simple descriptive-adjectives scales to detailed questionnaires assessing pain on different dimensions of pain experience (e.g. McGill Pain Questionnaire). Short descriptions of the main classifications of pain are given, and the patient is asked to indicate an appropriate phrase or number to describe his or her condition. Examples include the graphic verbal rating scale, the visual analogue scale and the numerical rating scale (Fig. 6.2).

• *Pain relief tools.* These are similar to pain measurement tools but assess the effect of analgesia given.

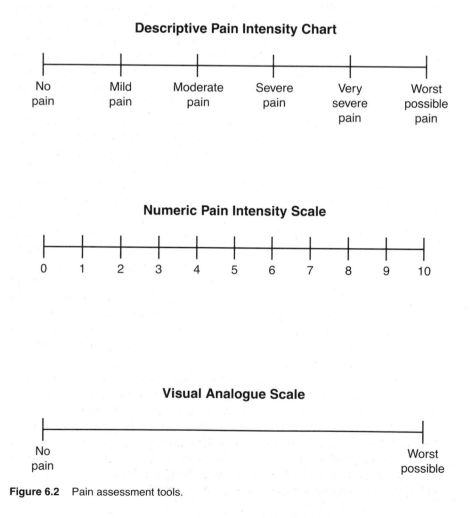

**Figure 6.2**   Pain assessment tools.

- *Tools to elicit nurse perception of patient pain*. Although measures have been devised to ascertain nurse perception of patient pain, they are time-consuming to complete and are of doubtful clinical value.

Barbonnais (1981) identified the following items as being essential in assessing patients' pain:

- knowledge of the patient's personal coping strategies
- observation and use of cues from the patient rather than waiting for the patient to request relief
- full understanding of the cause of pain
- careful observation of the patient's non-verbal behaviour
- recognising one's own bias.

A clear implication of this paper is that the assessment of the patient with respect to pain should begin long before the postoperative phase of management. This need has been highlighted in a study of 105 patients undergoing third molar surgery, in which their anxieties were assessed pre- and postoperatively (Earl 1994). Although 88% of these patients assessed their pain as better than expected, 43% rated it the factor they would fear most if the procedure were repeated. Obviously, pain is the single most feared factor despite evidence that it is usually no worse than originally feared.

The link between preoperative preparation of the patient in terms of expectations and coping strategies and the postoperative clinical course has been further explored by Vallerand et al (1994). Forty patients scheduled to undergo third molar surgery were randomly assigned to one of two groups. Treatment group members were given postoperative instructions that included descriptive information regarding potential sequelae (e.g. pain, oedema, trismus and nausea) as well as detailed information regarding analgesia use. Control group members were given basic open-ended postoperative wound care instructions. Postoperative pain and satisfaction with pain control were recorded using a visual analogue scale. Patients in the treatment group reported significantly less pain during the period 12–18 hours and 24 hours postoperatively, but there was no significant difference in analgesic consumption between the groups. These results suggest that increasing the quantity of postoperative preparatory information increases pain relief and resultant satisfaction with pain control without increasing analgesic consumption.

So much for pain assessment in adults. What about children? In some ways this may be easier because of their natural honesty and open expressions. On the other hand, one needs to be aware of the limitations of their language skills and their need to trust an adult before confiding in him or her.

The child under 2 may express pain through crying, increased irritability, head rolling, lethargy, flexing extremities, loss of appetite and loss of interest in play. Once a child is able to talk, the QUESTT tool is of considerable help in pain assessment (Whaley & Wong 1991):

- Question the child.
- *Use* pain rating slides.
- *E*valuate behaviour and physical changes.
- *S*ecure patient involvement.
- *T*ake cause of pain into account.
- *T*ake action and evaluate results.

Clearly it is advantageous to adapt the pain rating scales appropriately to the age of the child. Colour charts, cartoon type faces indicating smiling and grimacing, and simple linear scales have all been used successfully.

## PLANNING

In the introduction to this chapter it was established that, in general, nursing assessment of pain is often inadequate, and some of the possible reasons for this were mentioned. By implication, without a satisfactory method of assessment and an appropriate knowledge base, it is difficult to address the issue of planning for postoperative pain management. Sofaer (1985) details the need for a specific ward-based education programme to focus on the management of postoperative pain. At the national level the Royal College of Nursing's pain interest group outlines proposals for integrating a comprehensive pain management component into the existing registered general nurse educational curriculum (Davis & Seers 1991).

## IMPLEMENTATION

In simplified form the management of acute postoperative pain can be divided into treatment with either opiates or non-opiate preparations or indeed sometimes with a combination of both.

### Opiates

Opiates produce analgesia as a result of their agonist effects on receptors in the central nervous system. Effective doses can be administered by the oral, rectal, transdermal or sublingual routes or by subcutaneous, intramuscular or intravenous infusion or injection. Of these options, intramuscular opiates have been the most common treatment of choice for patients after surgery. This practice has been based on the apparent simplicity of the technique. A dose of opiate is often prescribed to be given as often as the doctor or nurse considers it to be necessary and safe. Unfortunately, the orders too frequently provide for a standard dose that is optimal only for a small range of patients, and the 'as necessary' part of the order is interpreted to mean 'as little as possible'. There is typically little flexibility in doses or injection intervals for individual patients. The resulting conservative prescriptions result in inadequate analgesia for many.

As we discussed in the introduction to this chapter, one reason for the nurse's reluctance to use opiates is the fear of untoward side effects. These are listed in Box 6.1.

### Administration of opiates

In most patients and in doses that have the same analgesic effect, the incidence of side effects is very similar regardless of the opiate used. The important principle to remember is that the safe and effective administration of opiates is a process of titration: for an opioid to be effective it must reach a certain concentration in the blood (the minimum effective analgesic concentration – MEAC). No pain relief is experienced below this level. Above it there is increasing analgesia and side effects are more likely.

Although patient age is the best clinical predictor of dose requirement the titration of sequential doses of opiate is determined by:

- the onset of action; this depends primarily on the route of administration – for morphine given intravenously this is about 15 minutes
- the duration of action; this depends on:
  - the amount given
  - the route of administration
  - the pharmacokinetics of the drug given
- the monitoring of pain scores, sedation scores and respiratory rate
- the occurrence of side effects.

---

**Box 6.1**   Side effects of opiates

- Respiratory
    Respiratory depression
- Neurological
    Sedation
    Euphoria/dysphoria
    Nausea and vomiting
    Miosis
    Muscle rigidity
- Cardiovascular
    Vasodilatation
    Bradycardia
    Myocardial depression
- Urinogenital
    Urinary retention
- Gastrointestinal
    Delayed gastric emptying
    Constipation
- Integumentary
    Pruritis

---

All opiates are capable of producing the same degree of pain relief if adjustments are made to dose and route of administration. Comparative doses are shown in Table 6.1. The different routes of administration can be discussed more easily after consideration of Figure 6.3.

### Systemic opiates

*Intramuscular opiates.* It can be seen from the graph in Figure 6.3 that if a 4-hourly regimen were followed, the patient would remain in pain for some 4 hours after the initial injection. The subsequent two doses would produce effective analgesia. From the fourth dose onwards, however, as well as achieving analgesia there would be an increase in the likelihood of side effects. Clearly, the aim should be to contain the 'peaks and troughs' within the analgesic corridor. Intramuscular administration fails to do this unless small doses are given very frequently, which is unpopular with both patients and staff.

*Intravenous opiates.* Intermittent doses of opiates via this route would lead to large variations in blood concentrations, with little time in the analgesic corridor, as seen in Figure 6.3 for intermittent intramuscular administration. Intravenous opiate infusions can abolish these wide swings and permit prompt titration of drug to individual needs. Accumulation may occur using drugs that have an intermediate or long half-life, necessitating ongoing assessment and adjustment of dose to meet changing needs. Respiratory depression of life-threatening severity has been reported, and, as mentioned earlier, concern for this risk has limited the widespread use of continuous opiate infusions for postoperative pain.

*Oral opiates.* Oral opiates in appropriate doses are remarkably effective. Their use after major maxillofacial procedures may be limited by the patient's difficulty in swallowing, resulting from the surgery itself. They can, however, be given as an elixir through a nasogastric or gastrostomy

**Table 6.1** Equianalgesic doses of some of the commonly used opioids

| Opioid | Route | |
|---|---|---|
| | IM/IV (mg) | Oral (mg) |
| Morphine | 10 | 30–60 |
| Pethidine | 100 | 400 |
| Papaveretum | 15 | – |
| Codeine | 130 | 200 |
| Fentanyl | 0.1 | – |
| Diamorphine | 5 | 60 |
| Methadone | 10 | 20 |
| Buprenorphine | 0.4 | 0.8[a] |
| Pentazocine | 40–60 | 150 |

[a] sublingual

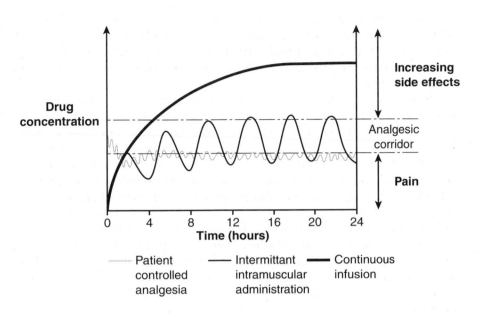

**Figure 6.3**   A comparison of different routes of opiate administration.

tube once postoperative ileus has resolved. If given before this the opiate can build up in the stomach and, when normal peristalsis resumes, a large bolus is transported to the large intestine where it is absorbed leading to overdose and unwanted side effects.

*Topical opiates.*  Traditionally, opiates are administered for the purpose of producing analgesia through their actions within the central nervous system. Studies examining their use at peripheral sites have produced conflicting results which have been reviewed previously (Stein 1993). Certainly no significant analgesic efficacy was found when morphine was placed in dental sockets after third molar surgery, albeit at relatively low dosages (Moore et al 1994).

**Patient-controlled analgesia (PCA).**  PCA, the self-administration of small doses of opiates by patients when they experience pain, was originally developed to minimise the effects of pharmacokinetic and pharmodynamic variability among individual patients. It is based on the premise that a negative feedback loop exists: when pain is experienced, analgesic medication will be demanded; when the pain is reduced, there will be no further demands.

Most intravenous PCA devices consist of a microprocessor-controlled pump triggered by depressing a button. When triggered, a pre-set amount (incremental dose) of opiate is delivered. A timer in the pump prevents administration of another bolus until a specified period has elapsed.

A considerable variety of devices for this purpose are now commercially available, and many offer the option to add a continuous background infusion to the basic patient-controlled mode.

The quality of analgesia with PCA has been consistently reported as superior or equal to that with intramuscular opiate. Less PCA opiate use compared with intramuscular control groups is frequently observed, and satisfaction of patients and nurses is high. The main advantages to patients of PCA are high-quality analgesia, autonomy, elimination of delay in decisions to medicate for pain, and freedom from painful intramuscular injections. Optimal efficacy and safety using PCA, as with other forms of treatment for postoperative pain, requires careful planning, establishment of appropriate policies and procedures and frequent medical assessment of the patient.

Side effects resulting from PCA include nausea, vomiting and itching and can be treated by changing the opiate in the pump or with drugs that provide symptomatic relief. The problem of vomiting is of particular concern in patients with potentially compromised airways, and to date the use of PCA following maxillofacial surgery has not been well received (Foley et al 1994).

## Non-opiate analgesia

*Non-steroidal anti-inflammatory drugs (NSAIDs)*

NSAIDs act principally through the inhibition of prostaglandin synthesis. Advantages over opiates include a reduction in opiate-related side effects, especially respiratory depression, absence of addiction potential and less sedation. A feared potential complication of NSAID administration is increased postoperative bleeding, especially into closed spaces. No data to indicate that this actually occurs in greater frequency with NSAID administration than without can be found in the literature.

Most evaluations of NSAIDs for postoperative pain relief have involved comparisons with opiates in 'either/or' protocols. With an improved understanding of postoperative pain and its consequences, there is growing emphasis on the advantages of combined approaches to therapy (Dahl et al 1990). Systemic opiates with centrally mediated actions and concurrent NSAIDs with peripheral sites of action appear to have advantages over either class of drug used alone. It is unlikely that NSAIDs can completely replace opiates in most patients suffering moderate and severe postoperative pain immediately after surgery (Ready 1994). In these cases, NSAIDs may best be considered as adjuncts to opiate therapy, with benefits that include a reduction in opiate requirements.

For many maxillofacial procedures, in particular the removal of third molars, NSAIDs alone are a very effective means of analgesia as well as when combined with steroids (Hersh et al 1993). There have been a number of comparative studies of various NSAIDs, with some conflicting reports, but, in general, diclofenac sodium has had the most favourable reviews, especially when given orally in a soluble form (Bailey et al 1993; Bakshi et al 1994). Diflunisal has also been shown to be effective and has a long duration of action (Lawton & Chapman 1993).

### Steroids

The use of corticosteroids in pain control after maxillofacial surgery has been reviewed, with the conclusion that their use in procedures other than third molar surgery needs more research (Gersema & Baker 1992). When given prophylactically, dexamethasone has been shown to significantly reduce postoperative pain and swelling and to eliminate the need for opiate analgesia (Baxendale et al 1993).

### Nitrous oxide

Under some circumstances, nitrous oxide ($N_2O$) can be a useful analgesic, especially for acutely painful experiences of short duration. Examples include repeated postoperative dressing changes or superficial wound debridement. The low solubility of nitrous oxide provides rapid onset of analgesia and rapid elimination on cessation of inhalation. Nitrous oxide in concentrations of 30–50% delivered through an anaesthetic machine or a calibrated mixer is said to be as potent as 10 mg of intramuscular morphine. The use of nitrous oxide in the UK is widespread, where it is available as a commercial 50% mixture with oxygen (Entonox).

## Local analgesia

Local anaesthetics are drugs which produce a transient and reversible loss of sensation in a circumscribed region of the body. Chemically, they are esters (procaine, amethocaine) or amides (lignocaine, prilocaine, bupivicaine), usually in the form of their acid salts. They act by preventing the initiation and propagation of nerve impulses by blocking the passage of sodium ions across the nerve cell membrane.

For many procedures (not those on the extremities) local anaesthetic agents are administered in combination with vasoconstrictors, for example, lignocaine 2% with adrenaline 1:80 000 is a common combination. The latter delays the absorption of the local anaesthetic, thus prolonging its action and reducing the side effects associated with rapid systemic absorption. When vasoconstrictor drugs are used, care must be taken, as they can affect the heart and circulation as well as reducing potassium levels. Hence caution must be exercised with general anaesthetics (halothane sensitises the heart to catecholamines), tricyclic antidepressants and potassium-loosing diuretics. In appropriate dosage felypressin is a suitable alternative vasoconstrictor.

*Administration of local anaesthetics*

Local anaesthetics can be administered topically, by infiltration or as regional blocks. Many head and neck procedures are carried out in this way, especially in general dental practice and outpatient clinics.

**Topical administration.** Various solutions, jellies, lozenges and sprays are frequently used in a number of ways; these are discussed in Chapter 3.

**Infiltration.** Infiltration involves injecting the local anaesthetic agent directly into the operative site, where it acts upon sensory nerve endings and small cutaneous nerves. This is particularly useful for dentoalveolar procedures in the upper jaw and for small procedures on the skin which do not justify a general anaesthetic. Infiltration to the surgical site, given intra-operatively, under general anaesthetic have been shown to reduce pain scores and analgesic requirements in the first postoperative day (Tuffin et al 1989), although less favourable results have been reported by Tordoff et al (1996). No significant differences in pain scores were observed at any stage between sites infiltrated with lignocaine and those with saline. Similar results were obtained in a study of tonsillectomy patients (Orntoft et al 1994).

The infusion of local anaesthetics into a wound site postoperatively has been recommended as a technique after harvesting of bone from the iliac crest or rib in various head and neck procedures. In this case, bupivicaine is infused into the donor site through an epidural cannula inserted into the operative site (Hahn et al 1995).

**Regional blockade.** Regional nerve blocks are given by injecting the local anaesthetic agent around a large branch of a nerve to anaesthetise a wide area peripheral to the injection site. Branches of the maxillary and mandibular division of the trigeminal nerve are amenable to nerve-blocking techniques. By far the most common block used is the inferior dental block, which anaesthetises the lower lip, mandible and lower teeth of one side as well as part of the oral mucosa.

## Other methods of pain control

*Transcutaneous electrical nerve stimulation (TENS)*

TENS is widely used in the management of chronic pain but can also be used to provide postoperative analgesia. The technique is simple, non-invasive and free of toxicity, although the mechanism by which analgesia is produced is not known. Patients receive information and instruction pre-operatively. Immediately after wound closure, sterile electrodes are applied to the skin on either side of the incision. The wound is dressed and the electrodes are connected to a stimulator which produces a vibrating, tingling, soothing sensation. Stimulation is started using predetermined settings with subsequent adjustments to produce maximum benefit. TENS has not been evaluated for specific head and neck procedures, and there is still considerable controversy regarding its general efficacy (Tyler et al 1982).

*Laser therapy*

Low level laser treatment after the removal of third molar teeth has been shown to be ineffective (Fernando et al 1993, Roynesdal et al 1993).

*Acupuncture*

In the one study in the current literature exploring this subject, acupuncture was given to two groups of patients undergoing the removal of third molar teeth. In one group it was given preoperatively, and in the other group it was given postoperatively. A control group received no acupuncture at all. Postoperatively patients in the two treatment groups reported higher pain levels than the control group. The reasons for this were not clear (Ekblom et al 1991).

## EVALUATION

Careful evaluation of pain management can only be carried out if we are prepared to make the tedious observations and recordings that are required. An example of an observation chart for opiate infusion is shown in Figure 6.4, but it must be remembered that evaluation is an ongoing process which takes the form of a feedback loop which may need to be repeated several times. Such loops are illustrated in Figures 6.5 and 6.6. Such algorithms are very useful and can be adapted to suit the circumstances of the individual hospital, unit or ward area.

The responsibility of developing appropriate protocols and educating both medical and nursing staff nowadays is often undertaken by the acute pain service. The first such service was started at the University of Washington in Seattle in 1986, and the concept has spread widely since. These multidisciplinary teams include a specialist nurse and are usually led by an anaesthetist. It is the way of the world that new ideas are difficult to implement, and gaining consensus from naturally conservative professionals may be seen as impossible. Nevertheless, the sharing of ideas from a number of interested parties can be stimulating and lead to improvements in pain control which are long overdue.

### PROTOCOL FOR USE OF POST-OPERATIVE INFUSION PUMPS

THE FOLLOWING ASSESSMENTS SHOULD BE USED TO RECORD PAIN, SEDATION AND VOMITING.

**PAIN SCORE**
0 = NO PAIN AT REST / MOVEMENT
1 = NO PAIN AT REST / SLIGHT PAIN ON MOVEMENT
2 = INTERMITTENT PAIN AT REST / MODERATE ON MOVEMENT
3 = CONTINUOUS PAIN AT REST / SEVERE ON MOVEMENT

**VOMITING SCORE**
0 = NIL
1 = NAUSEA
2 = VOMITING LAST HOUR

**SEDATION SCORE**
0 = NONE (patient alert)
1 = MILD (occasionally drowsy)
2 = MODERATE (frequently drowsy: easy to arouse)
3 = SEVERE (somnolent: difficult to arouse)
S = SLEEP (normal sleep: easy to arouse)

INITIAL RATE WILL BE DETERMINED IN THEATRE RECOVERY. THIS RATE SHOULD BE MAINTAINED FOR THE DURATION OF THE INFUSION: UNLESS

|   |   | **ACTION** |
|---|---|---|
| 1. | RESPIRATORY RATE <br> <12 | STOP INFUSION FOR 1 HOUR. <br> RESTART AT HALF PREVIOUS RATE. |
| 2. | RESPIRATORY RATE <br> <10 | STOP INFUSION. <br> AWAKEN PATIENT IF POSSIBLE. <br> CONTACT MO <br> (ANAESTHETIST IF AVAILABLE, SURGICAL IF NOT). |
| 3. | ANALGESIA INADEQUATE | CONTACT MO WHO MAY, AFTER SEEING THE PATIENT, GIVE A BOLUS DOSE OR INCREASE THE RATE OF INFUSION. |
| 4. | PATIENT BECOMES HYPOTENSIVE AND SHOCKED | CONTACT MO AND STOP INFUSION. |

**PATIENT MONITORING**
1.  ALL PATIENTS **MUST** HAVE ACCURATE HOURLY RESPIRATORY RATE. THIS WILL DETERMINE THE INFUSION RATE AS ABOVE.

2.  PATIENTS MUST BE NURSED IN HIGH DEPENDENCY AREA. (ELSEWHERE ONLY ON DIRECT RESPONSIBILITY OF CONSULTANT INITIATING INFUSION, AND FREQUENCY OF RESPIRATORY RATE MUST BE INCREASED TO HALF HOURLY).

3.  RATE OF ANALGESIC INFUSION IN ml/hour (3 FIGURES ON SYRINGE PUMP) =

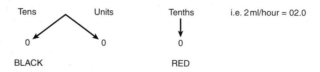

4.  AMOUNT OF INFUSION REMAINING IN SYRINGE SHOULD BE RECORDED AS WELL AS AMOUNT ADMINISTERED BY PATIENT WITH RATE OF INFUSION ON OBSERVATION CHART. THIS WILL PROVIDE MONITORING OF THE CORRECT FUNCTIONING OF THE SYRINGE PUMP AND PREVENT INADVERTENT UNDER OR OVERDOSE.

5.  RECORD ANY BOLUS IV DOSE GIVEN BY MO ON OBSERVATION CHART ALONGSIDE RESPIRATORY RATE. IM OPIATES MUST **NOT** BE GIVEN TO ANY PATIENT ON AN ANALGESIA INFUSION. THE COMBINATION MAY CAUSE SEVERE RESPIRATORY DEPRESSION.

**Figure 6.4**   Opiate infusion chart.

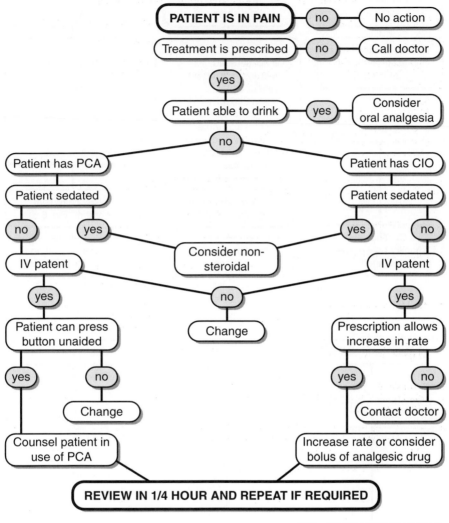

**Figure 6.5**   Pain relief algorithm.

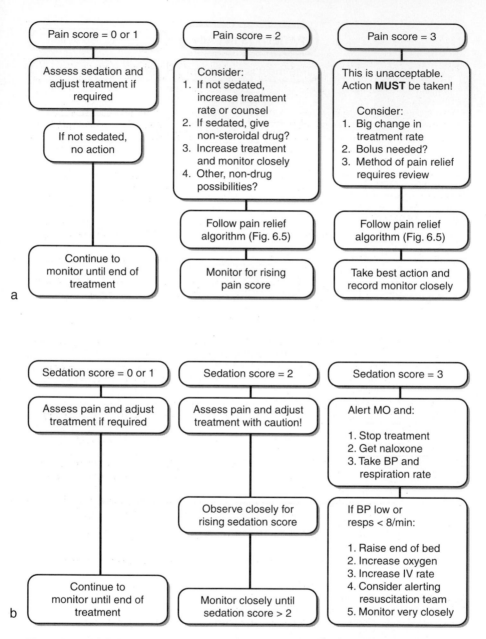

**Figure 6.6**   (a) Pain relief algorithm. (b) Sedation score algorithm. The pain relief and sedation score algorithms indicate possibilities; care must be taken to match actions against the patient's own physical, psychological and personal needs.

REFERENCES

Bailey B M, Zaki G, Rotman H, Woodwards R T 1993 A double-blind comparative study of soluble aspirin and diclofenac dispersible in the control of post-extraction pain after removal of impacted third molars. International Journal of Oral and Maxillofacial Surgery 22(4): 238–241

Bakshi R, Frenkel G, Dietlein G, Meurer-Witt B, Scheider B, Sinterhauf U 1994 A placebo-controlled comparative evaluation of diclofenac dispersible versus ibuprofen in post-operative pain after third molar surgery. Journal of Clinical Pharmacology 34(3): 225–230

Barbonnais F 1981 Pain assessment: development of a tool for the nurse and the patient. Journal of Advanced Nursing 6: 277–282

Baxendale B R, Vater M, Lavery K M 1993 Dexamethasone reduces pain and swelling following extraction of third molar teeth. Anaesthesia 48(11): 961–964

Caunt H 1992 Reducing the psychological impact of postoperative pain. British Journal of Nursing 1(1): 13–14

Commission on the Provision of Surgical Services 1990 Report of the Working Party on Pain after Surgery. Royal College of Surgeons of England and The College of Anaesthetists, London

Dahl J B, Rosenberg J, Dirks W E et al 1990 Prevention of post-operative pain by balanced analgesia. British Journal of Anaesthesia 64: 518

Davis P, Seers K 1991 Teaching nurses about managing pain. Nursing Standard 5(52): 30–32

Davitz L, Pendleton S 1969 Nurses inference of patient suffering. Nursing Research 18: 100–107

Earl P 1994 Patients' anxieties with third molar surgery. British Journal of Oral and Maxillofacial Surgery 32(5): 293–297

Ekblom A, Hansson P, Thomsson M 1991 Increased postoperative pain and consumption of analgesics following acupuncture. Pain 44(3): 241–247

Fernando S, Hill C M, Walker R 1993 A randomised double-blind comparative study of low level laser therapy following surgical extraction of third molar teeth. British Journal of Oral and Maxillofacial Surgery 31(3): 170–172

Foley W L, Edwards R C, Jacobs L F 1994 Patient controlled analgesia: a comparison of dosing regimens for acute postsurgical pain. Journal of Oral and Maxillofacial Surgery 52(2): 155–159

Gersema L, Baker K 1992 Use of corticosteroids in oral surgery. Journal of Oral and Maxillofacial Surgery 50(3): 270–277

Hahn M J, Dover M S, Whear N M, Mole I 1995 Local bupivicaine infusion following bone graft harvest from the iliac crest. International Journal of Oral and Maxillofacial Surgery 25(5): 400–401

Hersh E V, Cooper S, Betts N et al 1993 Single dose and multi-dose analgesic study of ibuprofen and meclofenamate sodium after third molar surgery. Oral Surgery, Oral Medicine, Oral Pathology 76(6): 680–687

Kitson A 1994 Postoperative pain management: a literature review. Journal of Clinical Nursing 3(1): 7–18

Kuhn S, Cook K, Collins M et al 1990 Perceptions of pain after surgery. British Medical Journal 300: 1687–1690

Lawton G M, Chapman P J 1993 Diflunisal – a long acting non-steroidal anti-inflammatory drug: a review of its pharmacology and effectiveness in the management of post-operative dental pain. Australian Dental Journal 38(4): 265–271

Mackintosh C 1994 Do nurses provide adequate post-operative pain relief? British Journal of Nursing 3(7): 343–347

Merskey H, Alse-Fessard D G, Bonica J J 1979 Pain terms: a list of definitions and notes on usage. Pain 6: 249

Moore U J, Seymour R A, Gilroy J, Rawlins M D 1994 The efficacy of locally applied morphine in post-operative pain after bilateral third molar surgery. British Journal of Clinical Pharmacology 37(3): 227–230

Orntoft M D, Longreen M D, Moiniche S et al 1994 A comparison of pre and post-operative tonsillar infiltration with bupivicaine for pain after tonsillectomy: a pre-emptive effect? Anaesthesia 94: 151–154

Ready L B 1994 Acute post-operative pain. In: Miller R D (ed) Anaesthesia, 4th edn. Churchill Livingstone, Edinburgh

Roynesdal A K, Bjornland T, Barkvoll P, Haanaes H R 1993 The effect of a soft laser application on post-operative pain and swelling: a double-blind study. International Journal of Oral and Maxillofacial Surgery 22(4): 242–245

Sofaer B 1985 Pain management through nurse education. In: Recent advances in nursing: perspectives on pain. Churchill Livingstone, Edinburgh

Stein C 1993 Peripheral mechanisms of opoid analgesia. Anaesthetic Analogue 76: 182

Tordoff J G, Brassy M, Rowbotham D J et al 1996 The effect of pre-incisional infiltration with lignocaine for post-operative pain after molar teeth extraction under general anaesthetic. Anaesthesia 51: 585–587

Tuffin J R, Cunliffe D R, Shaw S R 1989 Do local analgesics injected at the time of third molar removal under general anaesthesia, reduce significantly post-operative analgesic requirements? A double-blind controlled trial. British Journal of Oral and Maxillofacial Surgery 27: 27–32

Tyler E, Caldwell C, Ghia J N 1982 TENS: an alternative approach to the management of post-operative pain. Anaesthetic Analogue 61: 449

Vallerland W P, Vallerand A H, Heft M 1994 The effects of pre-operative preparatory information on the clinical course following third molar extraction. Journal of Oral and Maxillofacial Surgery 52(11): 1165–1170

Whaley L, Wong D 1991 Nursing care of infants and children. Mosby Year Book, St Louis

# 7

# Communication problems

'Speech is civilisation itself. The word, even the most contradictory word, preserves contact – it is silence which isolates'

Thomas Mann

---

KEY POINTS

- The processes of speech
- Hearing and speech assessment
- Aids to hearing and speech

---

## INTRODUCTION

The ability to communicate is a vital part of one's sense of identity. It is used to shape our environment, establish our position in society and to state our ideas, thoughts and emotions. Even the sound of our voice is part of our identity (Casper & Colton 1993). In particular, the absence of the ability to explain oneself, especially during a very difficult period, can cause or contribute to a sense of isolation and depression.

The management of problems resulting from a reduced ability to communicate in head and neck patients is a very specialised area. In most general hospital settings there is close liaison between the surgeons, nurses, audiologists and speech therapists in the care of such patients. Clearly it is beyond the remit of this book to deal with any of these specialties in depth, but it may be useful to outline some of the main aspects of care involved. For descriptive purposes we will deal with hearing and speech problems separately, although of course in reality the two are closely tied up with each other.

# ANATOMY AND PHYSIOLOGY
# Speech

Speech is the complex psychophysiological process by which sequences of sounds are selected to form words articulated within a grammatical framework. There are several requirements for normal speech development, including:

- adequate hearing
- stimulation from the environment
- maturation and correct functioning of the neuropsychological processes
- intelligence
- normal function of the pharynx and larynx
- emotional stability.

Most of these requirements have been dealt with elsewhere in this book. Two that need more attention are phonation and auditory feedback. In this section we will try to link them together to illustrate the high degree of integration required for effective communication.

## *Phonation*

Phonation is mediated by the larynx, which is a respiratory organ situated between the pharynx and the trachea. It lies below the hyoid bone in the midline of the neck, where the laryngeal prominence, or Adam's apple, is the most obvious part. It projects backwards into the pharynx and becomes continuous with the trachea at the level of the C6 vertebra.

The larynx is composed of several irregularly shaped cartilages attached to each other by ligaments and membranes (Figs 7.1 and 7.2). The main cartilages are as follows.

**The thyroid cartilage.** This consists of two flat pieces of hyaline cartilage, fused anteriorly, forming the laryngeal prominence. Immediately above this prominence the laminae are separated, forming a V-shaped notch known as the thyroid notch. The thyroid cartilage is incomplete posteriorly, and the posterior border of each lamina is extended to form the superior and inferior cornu (Fig. 7.3).

The upper part of the thyroid cartilage is lined with stratified squamous epithelium like the larynx, and the lower part with ciliated columnar epithelium like the trachea.

**The cricoid cartilage.** This lies below the thyroid cartilage and is composed of hyaline cartilage. It is shaped like a signet ring encircing the larynx, with the narrow band anteriorly. The broad posterior section articulates with the arytenoid cartilages above and the inferior cornu of the thyroid below (Fig. 7.4). It is lined with ciliated columnar epithelium.

**The arytenoid cartilages.** These are two pyramidal shaped cartilages situated on top of the broad part of the cricoid cartilage forming part of the posterior wall of the larynx. They give attachment to the vocal cords.

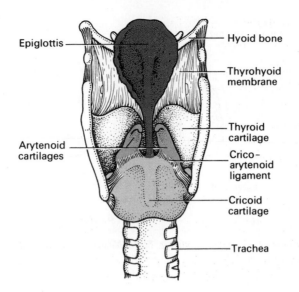

Epiglottis

Hyoid bone

Thyrohyoid membrane

Thyroid cartilage

Arytenoid cartilages

Crico-arytenoid ligament

Cricoid cartilage

Trachea

**Figure 7.1**   Larynx viewed from behind. From Wilson & Waugh 1996, with permission.

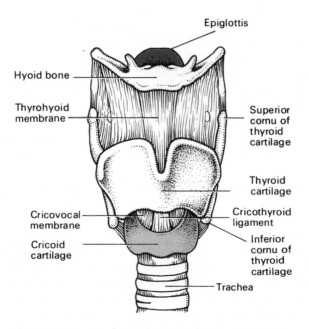

Epiglottis

Hyoid bone

Thyrohyoid membrane

Superior cornu of thyroid cartilage

Thyroid cartilage

Cricovocal membrane

Cricothyroid ligament

Inferior cornu of thyroid cartilage

Cricoid cartilage

Trachea

**Figure 7.2**   Larynx viewed from the front. From Wilson & Waugh 1996, with permission.

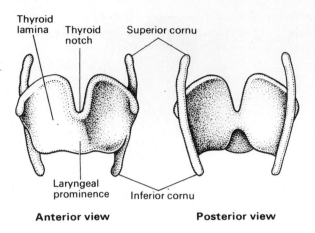

**Anterior view**          **Posterior view**

**Figure 7.3**   Thyroid cartilage. From Wilson & Waugh 1996, with permission.

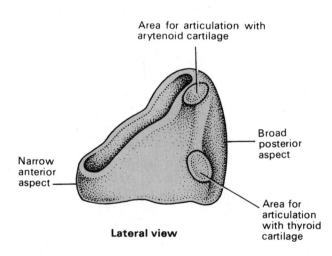

**Lateral view**

**Figure 7.4**   Cricoid cartilage. From Wilson & Waugh 1996, with permission.

**The epiglottis.** The epiglottis is a leaf-shaped fibroelastic cartilage attached to the inner surface of the anterior wall of the thyroid cartilage immediately below the thyroid notch. It rises obliquely upwards behind the tongue and the body of the hyoid bone. It is covered with stratified squamous epithelium.

The interior of the larynx comprises two groups of muscles: those that alter the size and shape of the inlet – the aryepiglottic, the oblique and transverse arytenoids – and those which move the vocal cords – the posterior and lateral cricoarytenoids, the thyroarytenoids, vocalis, transverse arytenoids and cricothyroids.

The vocal cords are two pale folds of mucous membrane with cord-like free edges which extend from the inner wall of the thyroid prominence anteriorly to the arytenoid cartilages posteriorly. The posterior cricoarytenoid is the single most important muscle in the larynx, and perhaps the body, as it is the only adductor of the vocal cords, which it achieves by rotating the arytenoid cartilages laterally. Contraction of the lateral cricoarytenoid muscles rotates the cartilages medially, pulling the cords together (Figs 7.5 and 7.6). When air is forced through the adducted cords they vibrate and sound is produced. These sounds are then manipulated by the tongue, cheeks and lips to produce speech.

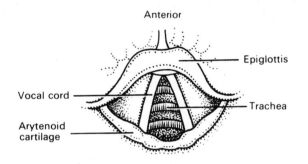

**Figure 7.5**    Interior view of the larynx viewed from above. From Wilson & Waugh 1996, with permission.

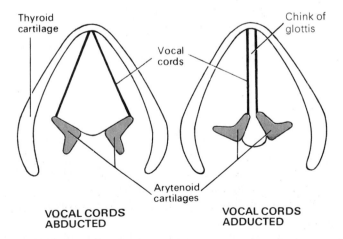

**Figure 7.6**    The extreme positions of the vocal cords. From Wilson & Waugh 1996, with permission.

Blood is supplied to the larynx by the superior and inferior laryngeal arteries and drained by the thyroid veins into the internal jugular vein.

All the muscles of the larynx are supplied by the recurrent laryngeal nerve except cricothyroid, which is supplied by the external laryngeal nerve.

## Articulation

The manipulation of the sound produced by the larynx is carried out by the tongue, soft palate, pharynx and the facial muscles. The anatomy of the first three of these organs has already been discussed in Chapter 3. The facial muscles involved in articulation are those of the lips and cheeks, but because of their importance in communication as a whole and their close relationship to speech, the muscles of the face need to be considered as a unit.

Functionally, the muscles of the face are differentiated to form groups around the orifices: the orbit, nose and mouth are guarded by the eyelids, nostrils and lips, and there is a sphincter and dilator arrangement peculiar to each. These muscles are sometimes referred to as the muscles of facial expression, but it is important to remember that facial expression is a learned characteristic: some of the muscles supplied by the facial nerve are incapable of affecting the expression of the face. Moreover, certain facial expressions are produced by muscles not supplied by the facial nerve: for example, levator palpebrae superioris, ocular muscles and the tongue.

**Muscles of the lips and cheeks.**

*Orbicularis oris.* This muscle forms the sphincter of the mouth cavity and consists of fibres encircling the cavity attached near the midline to the upper and lower jaws. Fibres from the dilator muscles (the remainder of the facial muscles) insert into these fibres. The nerve supply is by the buccal and marginal mandibular branches of the VIIth nerve. Contraction of orbicularis oris causes pursing of the lips.

*Buccinator.* This is the main muscle of the cheek, having a bony origin from both jaws opposite the molar teeth. It is essentially an accessory muscle of mastication, being indispensable to the return of the bolus from the cheek pouch to the molars. When the cheeks are puffed out the muscle is relaxed; contraction obliterates the cheek cavity and pulls the closed lips tightly back against the teeth. It is supplied by the VIIth nerve.

**The facial nerve.** The VIIth cranial nerve emerges from the base of the skull through the stylomastoid foramen and soon enters the parotid gland from which it emerges as five main groups of branches. The distribution of these branches can be outlined by placing the heel of the hand over the parotid gland, thumb on the temple and little finger down the neck. They comprise the following.

*Temporal branches.* These supply auricularis anterior and superior and part of frontalis. They are important in wrinkling the forehead.

*Zygomatic branches.* These consist of upper and lower branches which proceed above and below the eye. The upper branches supply frontalis and the upper part of orbicularis oculi. They cross the zygomatic arch and may be divided in incisions for operations on the temporal fossa, or injured in fractures of the zygomatic arch. The lower branches supply the lower half of orbicularis oculi and the muscles below the orbit. Two or three branches pass to both upper and lower eyelids. Damage to these prevents blinking, tears no longer spread, and the cornea quickly dries and ulcerates. The resultant scarring can impair vision.

*Buccal branches.* These supply buccinator and the fibres of the upper lip. Paralysis prevents emptying of the cheek pouch.

*Marginal mandibular branch.* This supplies the muscles of the lower lip. It emerges from the lower border of the parotid gland, and in 20% of cases passes into the neck below the angle of the mandible. It crosses the inferior border of the jaw to reach the face beyond the anterior border of masseter, crossing the facial artery and vein. A small lymph node lies here, and the nerve is in danger when incisions are made to drain infections within the node, as it is when submandibular incisions are made.

*Cervical branch.* This branch passes vertically downwards from the lower border of parotid, behind the mandible and supplies platysma.

## Auditory feedback

The organ of hearing is the ear, which for descriptive purposes is divided into three parts as follows.

*External ear*

This consists of the pinna and the external acoustic meatus (auditory canal) (Fig. 7.7). The former is a fibroelastic cartilaginous structure covered in skin, projecting from the side of the head. It has a lower lobular section composed of fibrous and adipose tissue.

The auditory canal is a slightly S-shaped tube about 2.5 cm long extending inwards from the pinna to the tympanic membrane. The lateral third is cartilaginous, and the middle third is in bone. It is lined with skin continuous with that of the pinna. In the lateral third the skin has numerous sebaceous and ceruminous (wax) glands.

The tympanic membrane separates the outer and middle ear. It is oval-shaped and made up of three types of tissue:

- an outer covering of hairless skin
- a middle layer of fibrous tissue
- an inner lining of mucous membrane continuous with that of the middle ear.

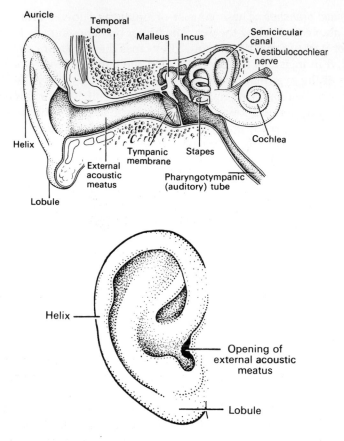

**Figure 7.7**   Pinna and external acoustic meatus. From Wilson & Waugh 1996, with permission.

## Middle ear (tympanic cavity)

This is an irregularly shaped cavity within the petrous section of the temporal bone. The cavity, its contents and the air sacs which open out of it are lined with simple squamous or cuboidal epithelium. The air reaches the cavity through the pharyngotympanic or Eustachian tube from the nasopharynx. The presence of air at atmospheric pressure on both sides of the tympanic membrane is maintained by the pharyngotympanic tube and enables the membrane to vibrate when sound waves strike it.

Extending across the middle ear cavity from the tympanic membrane to the oval window on the medial wall are three small bones: the malleus, incus and stapes (Fig. 7.8). These form a series of movable joints with each other and the medial wall, being held together by fine ligaments.

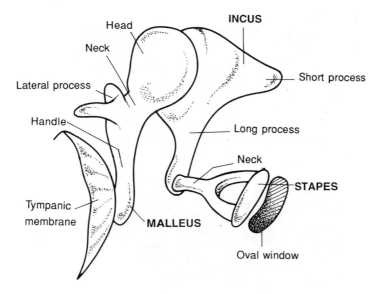

**Figure 7.8**  Malleus, incus and stapes. From Wilson & Waugh 1996, with permission.

*Internal ear*

This is a cavity in the temporal bone, lined with periosteum, containing the organs of hearing and balance. It has two parts: the bony labyrinth and the membranous labyrinth.

**Bony labyrinth.** This is larger than and encloses the membranous labyrinth, of the same shape, which fits into it (Fig. 7.9). Between the two there is a watery fluid called perilymph, and within the membranous labyrinth there is a similarly watery endolymph. The bony labyrinth is made up of the following.

*Vestibule.* This is the expanded part near the middle ear containing the oval and round windows.

*Cochlea.* This resembles a snail's shell. It has a broad base where it is continuous with the vestibule and a narrow apex.

*Semicircular canals.* These are three tubes arranged so that each is situated in one of the three planes of space. They are continuous with the vestibule.

**Membranous labyrinth.** As mentioned before, this is the same shape as its bony counterpart. A cross-section shows it to be triangular in shape (Fig. 7.10). Neuroepithelial cells and their nerve fibres lie on the basilar membrane and form the spiral organ of Corti, the peripheral sensory organ that responds to vibration by initiating nerve impulses, eventually perceived as hearing by the brain. The nerve fibres combine to form the auditory part of the vestibulo-cochlear or VIIIth cranial nerve, which passes through a foramen in the temporal bone to reach the hearing area in the temporal lobe of the cerebrum.

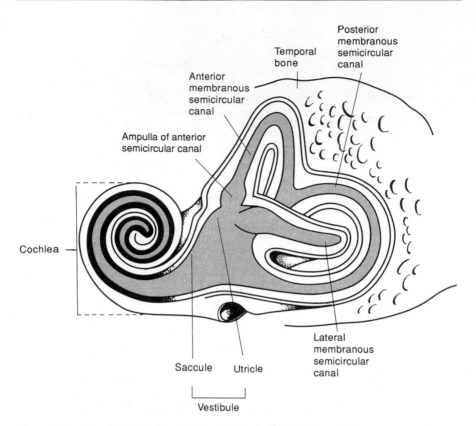

**Figure 7.9**  Bony labyrinth. From Wilson & Waugh 1996, with permission.

*Transduction of sound*

How then does hearing come about? Every sound produces sound waves or vibrations in the air which travel at about 332 m/s. These waves have properties of pitch and volume. Pitch is determined by the frequency of the sound waves and is measured in hertz (Hz). The volume, or intensity, depends upon the amplitude of the sound waves and is measured in decibels (dB).

The pinna concentrates the waves and directs them along the external auditory meatus, causing the tympanic membrane to vibrate. These vibrations are transmitted mechanically through the middle ear by the movements of the ossicles. At their medial end the footplate of the stapes rocks in the oval window and sets up fluid waves in the perilymph. These indent the membranous labyrinth, causing a wave motion in the endolymph, which stimulates the neuroepithelial cells of the spiral organ, and nerve impulses are generated as described above. The fluid wave is finally expended into the middle ear by vibration of the membrane around the round window.

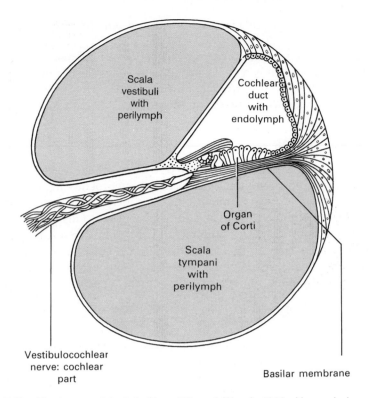

**Figure 7.10**    Membranous labyrinth. From Wilson & Waugh, 1996 with permission.

## ASSESSMENT
### Speech problems

The assessment of speech problems has two main components. Firstly, a case history and orofacial examination is undertaken, including an assessment of any dental prostheses that the patient may already use. Secondly, conventional voice laboratory baseline values are obtained, including frequency and intensity (acoustic) measurements, aerodynamic measurements and perceptual voice ratings. During the voice laboratory assessment, selective procedures focus on determining which techniques facilitate improvements in the voice.

Generally, facilitation approaches that probe the patient's respiratory support for voice and alter glottal attack, pitch and intensity can be initiated best using biofeedback. One can view the respiratory cycle using an oscilloscope or visualise phonation frequency with a Visi-pitch (Kay Elemetrics Corporation, Lincoln Park, NJ, USA) or other real time instrument. This visual feedback allows the patient to develop a feel for the level of respiratory and laryngeal effort required to produce improvement in the voice.

Use of audiotape recordings can increase auditory feedback of vocal production. The best voice can be recorded and played back to the patient, who must then learn to discriminate auditorily his or her best voice and to reproduce it with the least amount of effort.

## Hearing problems

Hearing loss is divided into bone conductive (sensorineural) and air conductive loss. The two most common forms of sensorineural hearing loss are presbycusis – a slow, progressive, initially high frequency loss that results from ageing changes within the inner ear – and noise-induced loss, such as industrial or occupational deafness. Conductive hearing loss can result either from fluid in the middle ear or from a problem with the ossicular chain.

In terms of service provision, Brooks (1989) suggested that it is important to have information about degree of hearing loss, as rehabilitation needs tend to increase with increasing severity. Overall, an individual's hearing ability can be measured by pure tone threshold audiometry and speech audiometry.

Hearing assessment can include self assessment by the individual and objective measures such as pure tone audiometry, in which sounds are produced at a known frequency. A pure tone sound can be quantified objectively by its intensity, which is measured in decibels (dB), and by its frequency, which is measured in hertz (cycles per second). These two parameters are perceived subjectively as loudness and pitch, respectively (Hawkes et al 1990). The sounds and intensity can be altered by the examiner.

The extent and cause of hearing loss can usually be determined from an examination of the audiogram (Fig. 7.11). For clinical purposes the range of normality is usually regarded as within 10 dB of the threshold of hearing impairment. Severity of hearing loss is determined by averaging the air conduction thresholds obtained at 500, 1000 and 2000 Hz. The degree of difficulty that an individual is likely to experience in understanding conversation can be determined by a speech discrimination scale. Brooks (1989) proposes, however, that a level which reflects difficulty in social communication is more appropriate than a statistically derived cut-off point. Additionally, with increasing age there exists a tendency to accept less acute hearing as an inevitable occurrence, a normal feature of ageing.

## PLANNING
## Speech problems

We have already established that pathology and surgery in the head and neck region can have a profound effect on speech. As we also know in gen-

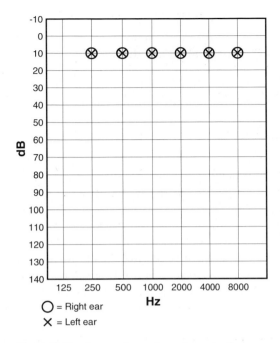

**Figure 7.11**   A normal pure tone air conduction audiogram.

eral terms what effects various surgical procedures have on speech, some degree of planning is possible. It almost goes without saying that the management of a very young child with a cleft lip and palate will be very different from that of an older patient after a major head and neck resection. Even within this latter group, however, it is not always possible to predict which patients will have what degree of difficulty postoperatively. Some of the commoner procedures and their effects are listed below.

*Mandibulectomy*

Resection of many oral carcinomas often necessitates removal of a significant section of the lower jaw. As many of the muscles involved in speech attach to the mandible, altered speech is almost inevitable postoperatively. Apart from the obvious need for early involvement of the speech therapist, a significant contribution can be made by the restorative dentist, who can provide appropriate prosthetic care ranging from conventional dentures to advanced crown and bridge work, often supported by osseointegrated implants.

*Maxillectomy*

The effect of tumours in this area on speech varies from minimal to quite severe and is highly dependent on the location of the tumour and the extent of the excision.

Tumours involving the alveolar ridge of the hard palate may result in a change in vocal resonance and distortion of some speech sounds. Tumours involving the soft palate will have a severe effect on vocal resonance and on the ability to produce many speech sounds – in which case, speech may be unintelligible (Casper & Colton 1993). Individuals following resection of the maxilla without placement of an obturator have deficits in speech resulting in hypernasal speech. This effect has been shown to be greatly diminished by placement of an obturator prosthesis (Kornblith et al 1996).

*Glossectomy*

Although there are several articulators used during the production of speech, the tongue is the most important. It is active during the production of all vowels and most of the consonants. Variation of tongue position in the anteroposterior dimension and in the cranial–caudal dimension is very apparent during the production of vowels to produce the appropriate reso-nance changes. Speech is affected by the mobility of the tongue, scars within the tongue itself, loss of volume due to degree of resection, loss of sensitivity and also displacement of the tongue by the bulk of soft tissue resection. How severely intelligibility is reduced depends on the extent of tongue removal and the ability of the patient to manipulate the remaining portion (Casper & Colton 1993; Kwakman et al 1997).

*Laryngectomy*

After the removal of the larynx, the individual no longer has a source of sound for speaking, and assistance with voice production is always required.

## Hearing problems

Hearing loss can result from a number of factors, such as impaction of wax in the external canal, trauma, congenital atresia, furuncles, otitis externia, middle ear disease, inclusive of acute otitis media, suppurative otitis media, Eustachian tube dysfunction, and a variety of drugs can cause audi-tory damage.

The successful management of any patient with a disorder of the ear demands both the ability to arrive at an adequate diagnosis and an under-standing of the medical and surgical principles of treatment. The broad aim of any treatment regime is to bring rapid symptomatic relief and to institute specific measures which will halt the disease process, thereby encouraging hearing and the restoration of normal structure and function. However the specific goals in managing a diseased ear are to achieve a safe, dry, symptom-free ear with good hearing and normal vestibular function (Hawkes et al 1990).

Effective planning for individuals with hearing impairment is aided by the fact that, on assessing results of the audiogram, trends are diagnostically supportive. For although, in purely sensorineural hearing loss, air and bone conductive thresholds will be the same, different specific patterns can be identified in the shape of the audiogram. For instance in presbyacusis the lower frequencies are usually normal, but in the higher frequencies the audiogram slopes downwards (Fig. 7.12). With noise-induced hearing loss, the deficit is maximal at 4000 Hz (Fig. 7.13a, b).

An additional important factor when planning care is that when examining air conductive hearing loss, if there are no external canal causative factors, it is important that middle ear function is assessed. As the clinical appearance of the tympanic membrane does not allow discrimination between fluid in the middle ear and problems with the ossicular chain, a tympanometry is required. This allows measurement of the mobility of the

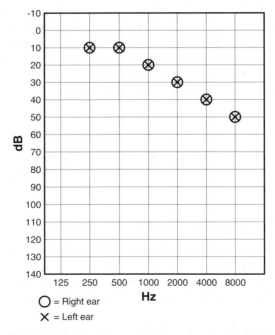

**Figure 7.12** Presbyacusis – a pure tone audiogram showing the typical high frequency sensorineural hearing loss that develops in some individuals with ageing.

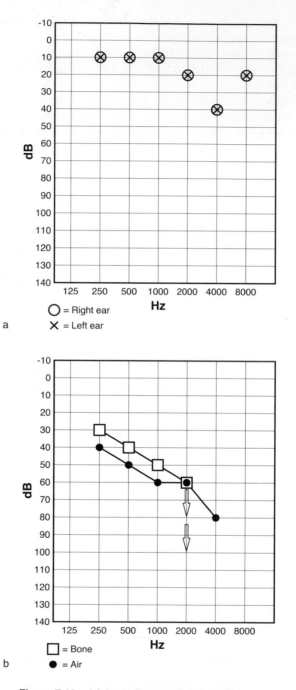

**Figure 7.13** (a) An audiogram showing noise-induced sensorineural hearing loss. (b) An audiogram showing sensorineural hearing loss.

tympanic membrane and pressure within the middle ear. Assessment of the results will allow for identification of the cause:

- fluid in the ear – the tympanogram tracing is flat (Fig. 7.14a)
- ossicular chain damage – the tympanogram tracing will peak to the left (Fig. 7.14b).

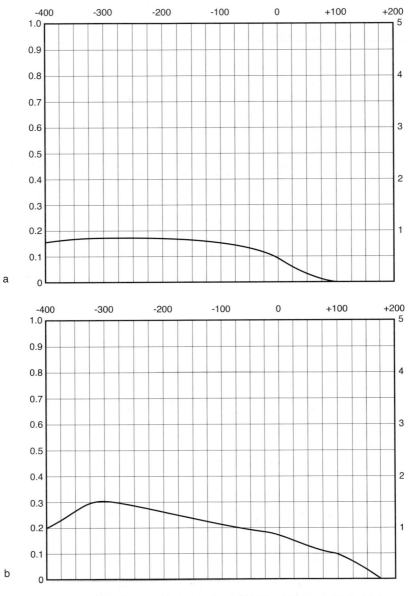

**Figure 7.14**   (a) A tympanogram demonstrating fluid in the middle ear (flat). (b) A tympanogram showing ossicular chain damage (peak shifted to the left).

# IMPLEMENTATION
## Speech problems
*Mandibulectomy*

When a tumour is located in and restricted to a portion of the mandible, and excision of only a portion of the mandible is indicated, the effects on speech are minimal. The individual often makes appropriate compensations spontaneously. Various forms of surgical reconstruction may be used, as well as prosthetic devices. Tumours that are more extensive, however, may involve portions of the tongue and floor of the mouth, thus increasing the likelihood of speech problems (Casper & Colton 1993).

*Maxillectomy*

Patients with alveolar ridge or hard palate defects are usually assessed for an intraoral prosthesis prior to surgery, and the prosthesis is inserted at the time of surgery. This is a temporary arrangement to allow healing to take place before the restorative dentist plans and provides the definitive prosthesis. Any minor speech problems remaining can usually be addressed through adaptation and habituation of compensatory behaviours.

Fitting of a prosthesis following excision of a soft palate tumour is more complex. A temporary prosthesis, without an obturating bulb extension, should be placed at the time of surgery. When healing has occurred, the prosthesis may be altered to include an obturating bulb (Casper & Colton 1993).

*Glossectomy*

Kwakman et al (1997) indicate that reconstructive surgery itself can impede speech. It is advantageous, therefore, that mobility of the tongue be improved as much as possible. Mobilising scar fixation of the base of the tongue from the mandible gives greater flexibility to the tongue. Additionally, Schliephake et al (1995) state that postoperative analysis of patients has shown that jejunal grafts are best in the lateral part of the mouth and have shortcomings in anterior locations.

Alternatively a prosthesis placed appropriately in the oral cavity can, with consideration for swallowing, improve the speech production abilities of individuals with total or partial glossectomy. A prosthesis may affect speech production abilities in different ways, however, depending on the amount of residual mass, mobility of the tongue and the extent of surgery. A prosthesis must be fashioned according to the unique needs and capabilities of the individual. Again, individuals with little tongue mass may have to develop compensatory movements to produce appropriate acoustics (Casper & Colton 1993).

## Pharyngolaryngectomy

Following pharyngolaryngectomy the convolutions intrinsic in the tissue are very different from the normal, relatively smooth-walled repaired pharynx with a vibrating pharyngo-oesophageal segment. Possibly because of the convolutions and the lack of muscle in the wall of the jejunum, leading to hypotonicity, combined with the fact that the pharynx is inverted and the jejunum is not, individuals repaired with jejunum have difficulty in generating sufficient voice to extend beyond one or two syllables per air change, even with the aid of digital pressure, resulting in virtual aphonia.

## Laryngectomy

Total laryngectomy as treatment for cancer of the larynx substantially alters speech. Subsequently the development of effective alaryngeal speech is a major step in rehabilitation of a laryngectomy patient. Current methods of vocal rehabilitation following laryngectomy include development of oesophageal speech, the use of the artificial larynx and, more recently, surgical restoration of voice.

**Oesophageal speech.** In this method of speech production, the vicarious air chamber is located within the body of the oesophagus. The neoglottis, or the pharyngo-oesophgeal (PE) segment, is located above the air chamber. The PE constriction is the vibratory site for production of oesophageal voice. Oesophageal speech uses regurgitation of swallowed air to produce vibration of the PE segment and hence sound, which is modified by the mouth, lips and tongue to produce the spoken word (Heaton & Parker 1994). It is noteworthy that a higher pressure is required to initiate and sustain vibrations in the PE segment than in the vocal folds (Debruyne et al 1994). There are two techniques for obtaining an air supply to inject from the mouth into the oesophagus via the tongue and the pharynx. The first of these involves two stages. Firstly, the tongue pushes air in the mouth back to the pharynx (the so-called glossal press). Secondly, the back of the tongue and pharynx force the air down into the oesophagus. These movements must be coordinated smoothly.

The second method involves inhalation. The patient must lower the pressure within the oesophageal segment relative to the atmospheric pressure. This permits air to flow from the outside (or inside the mouth) to the lower than normal pressure area in the oesophagus. To accomplish this, the patient must be able to relax the PE segment, otherwise air cannot flow downward. The forces that are responsible for the inhalation (and exhalation) of the air within the thorax also help in the 'inhalation' (and exhalation) of air from the oesophagus (Casper & Colton 1993).

Laryngectomy patients vary in their capacity to acquire a functional level of oesophageal speech. For although the basic attributes of oesophageal speech are now more clearly understood, substantial numbers of patients fail to develop functionally serviceable speech despite adequate therapy. The view that differences in function of the PE segment would be expected to influence the acquisition and development of serviceable oesophageal and tracheo-oesophageal speech is widely held by clinicians and researchers in the fields of surgery and speech pathology.

During speech the sphincter at the upper end of the oesophagus is in a constant state of activity, and the modulations of speech cause rapid variations in its tightness. The musculature of the upper oesophageal segment provides tone for the apposition of the mucosal surfaces and, in doing so, regulates airflow and serves as a source of sound generation. Following tumour removal surgeons strive to reconstruct the PE zone in a way such that the likelihood of alteration in oesophageal function is decreased. The surgical result therefore, seems to be a critical factor in the production of serviceable speech. Additionally, neural control of the PE zone is also a critical factor to be considered when interpreting the results of surgery (Sloane et al 1991).

Isshiki & Snidecor (1965) identified that air volume *per se* is not related to oesophageal speech proficiency, but that the air flow rates at exsufflation are important. Additionally the amount of tone supplied by the neoglottis or PE segment is one of the most important factors that affect air flow rate. McIvor et al (1990) noted that the volume of air which can be retained in the dilated oesophagus rarely exceeds 80 mL, and this tends to produce short phrases of quiet, low-pitched speech.

Hypotonicity, hypertonicity, spasm and stricture of the PE segment have all been shown to be detrimental to the production of oesophageal voice (McIvor et al 1990, Sloane et al 1991). Hypopharyngeal stricture is treated by dilatation; spasm in the PE segment is traditionally treated via myotomy. In addition, transcutaneous injection of botulinum toxin into the PE segment after laryngectomy has been shown to improve speech (Crary & Glowasky 1996).

**Mechanical vibrator speech.** Until recently the artificial larynx was considered to be the method of choice only for those patients who were unable to learn oesophageal speech. Many clinicians assumed that if the larynx was introduced before oesophageal speech training, the acquisition of oesophageal speech would be negated by the ease of using the artificial larynx. There does not seem to be any strong evidence that this is so, and, in any event, this may be the only method of acquiring alaryngeal speech for some patients. Some of the benefits of an artificial larynx include immediately and relatively intelligible speech, even while hospitalised, thereby reducing the frustration of having to communicate by writing. It also acts as temporary alternative for oesophageal speakers who experience fatigue, have upper respiratory tract infection or experience states of high emotion.

In mechanical vibrator speech a hand-held machine is placed in contact with the soft tissues of the neck to transmit vibrations to the floor of the mouth, and the individual uses the articulator, tongue, lips and soft palate to create speech from the artificial 'voice'. Various machines have been designed over the years but the established types in use today are simple vibrators. Most are electronic and have a manually adjustable fundamental frequency. These are typically set to a low pitch for a male voice and, where possible, to a higher value for a female voice. Users of an electrolarynx (Fig. 7.15) can produce average intensity levels during speech, typical of normal speech during ordinary conversation (Casper & Colton 1993, Heaton et al 1996).

**Tracheo-oesophageal speech.** The tracheo-oesophageal puncture method, coupled with the use of a voice prosthesis, was introduced nearly two decades ago (Singer & Blom 1980). Currently it is the surgical method of choice. This method of speech uses the natural air reservoir of the lungs. Surgical procedures have been devised to divert air from the trachea into the reconstructed pharyngo-oesophagus and thus increase the air flow through the PE segment (McIvor et al 1990). Air is redirected through the PE segment via a surgically created tracheo-oesophageal fistula. Such fistulas alone are prone to leakage and aspiration of saliva and other fluids into the lungs, or to closure by unwanted healing. A valved prosthesis was therefore developed (Fig. 7.16) which could be passed through the surgically created fistula between the trachea and pharynx, thereby allowing pulmonary air to be directed into the oesophagus for phonation, but closing at all other times to prevent aspiration (McIvor et al 1990, Heaton and Parker 1994). Leder & Erskine (1997) showed that tracheo-oesophageal tract stabilisation occurs over a period of 1 month after surgery, indicating that routine resizing of a valve fitted within this period is required.

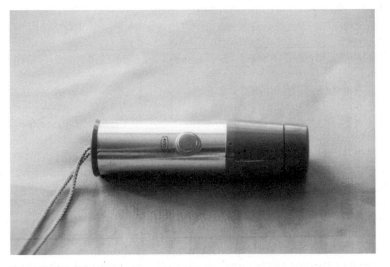

**Figure 7.15**   Electrolarynx.

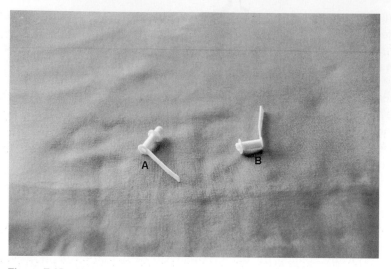

**Figure 7.16**   Valved prosthesis: A, Blom-Singer duckbill type; B, Blom-Singer low pressure type.

A major advantage of this approach is that the surgery is feasible in most patients who have had a laryngectomy, including those who have had radical neck dissection or those who have received radiotherapy. A second advantage is that the procedure is reversible. Furthermore, aspiration, which complicated earlier tracheo-oesophageal shunt procedures, is eliminated. This is not to say patients do not encounter leakage either around or through the prosthesis, but the rate is estimated to be less than 10% (Izdebski et al 1994). A final advantage is the rapid and successful acquisition of laryngeal speech with excellent fluency and intelligibility. Acoustic aerodynamic and intelligibility studies have shown that this type of speech is most often equal to or exceeds the best oesophageal speech (Williams & Watson 1985; Pindzola & Cain 1988).

Since the introduction of these devices, there have been several changes in design aimed at making them more anatomically compatible, more effective and easier to insert. Although the most recent indwelling prostheses allow extended wear, there remains the need, as with most prostheses, to train the patient in their care and use (Leder & Erskine 1997).

Contraindications for placement of a prosthesis include inability to care for the stoma, poor manual dexterity, a stenotic stoma and poor motivation. The development of the indwelling vocal prosthesis allows some people with poor manual dexterity or poor eyesight to achieve tracheo-oesophageal prosthetic speech as long as a carer can assist with cleansing the prosthesis.

This technique was initially introduced as a secondary procedure, but in recent years primary voice restoration, using the same technique, has been carried out at the same time as the laryngectomy. Some studies have shown that the primary procedure is as effective as, if not more so than, the secondary procedure.

## Hearing problems

Specific treatments for ear disease will not be discussed within the format of this book, as this topic is more than adquately covered in other text-books. It is important to remember, however, that the specific goals in managing a diseased ear are to achieve a safe, dry, symptom-free ear.

The majority of individuals with hearing impairment are able to communicate effectively. There are those who in order to function fully in everyday life will require some form of aural rehabilitation. This can incorporate the fitting of a hearing aid, assistive devices, speech reading and auditory training.

Most hearing aids are worn either in the ear or behind the ear. The most common are worn in the ear and consist of an ear mould which sits in the conchal bowl, extending into the outer part of the ear canal. These aids are relatively inconspicuous and are advantageous in that the microphone is able to pick up sounds fairly naturally, as unwanted sounds from behind the head are blocked by the pinna. Alternatively an aid worn behind the ear has the advantage of more electronics being fitted and therefore producing a more sophisticated device. Another aid which is more powerful than the previous two is the body aid. Unfortunately these are obtrusive and patient acceptance is poor. Consequently, they tend to be given only to those who are severely hard of hearing. One overall disadvantage of hearing aids is that they make all sounds louder, amplifying background noise as well as speech.

Assistive devices are classified into several categories including assistive listening devices, such as personal amplifiers, alerting devices incorporating loud bells and buzzers, signalling devices such as flashing lights and vibrating devices. Telecommunication devices such as computers with modems, and informing devices including captions for television may aid the hearing-impaired individual.

Speech reading may be relied upon; this is related to lip movement, grasping meaning as a whole rather than trying to decipher each specific element. In order for an individual to be competent, it is important that he or she is able to fill in gaps in the information flow. A factor for consideration in assessing the merits of combined auditory and visual input is the quality of the visual stimulus and the environmental situation in which speech reading is taking place. Lip-reading classes have been identified as beneficial in terms of improved self esteem, confidence and morale (Brooks 1989).

Auditory training describes the process where repeated exposure to auditory stimuli allows the individual to make better use of residual hearing. It allows enhancement of awareness and discrimination (Cahart 1961).

Another problem is that many communication situations are filled with distractions that can seriously interfere with the listening process. The effects of unwanted background noise, distance from the source of the sound, or poor room acoustics can create an insurmountable obstacle for the hearing impaired. In response to these problems a series of electronic devices have been developed which can improve the ability of the hearing-impaired person to communicate in specific listening situations. This, for example, includes the loop system by which, in places such as churches or cinemas, the hearing-impaired individual is assisted in establishing a means of effective hearing.

## EVALUATION

Historically the intent of treatment has been curative, and health care providers have focused their attention on outcome measures such as tumour response, disease-free survival, overall survival and control of major physical symptoms. Recently, however, there has been increasing interest in the behavioural and functional impact on the individual. There has also been increasing awareness of the need for patient reporting of these variables. This need has been emphasised by the studies in oncology that have shown physician and patient perceptions of clinical outcomes to be poorly correlated (D'Antonio et al 1996). In assessing alaryngeal speech, for example, a study by Heaton et al (1996) reported that higher scores were assigned by health professionals than by the patient. The high score recorded by the speech and language therapist was viewed as possibly resulting from their involvement with individuals with other voice problems, whereas a lower score by the patient may be because they can only compare themselves with the normal healthy population.

Acceptability judgements have been found to be based on clarity of articulation, amount of extraneous noise such as respiratory noise, appearance of confidence and casualness, coordination of speech with breathing, duration of sentences, retention of local accent and use of gestures. Clements et al (1997) suggest that research during the 1990s, although focusing on the effectiveness and intelligibility of the various methods of communication, has not directly addressed the individual's satisfaction with these and their effect on quality of life. Colangelo et al (1996) identified considerable deterioration in communication and understanding occurring in the preoperative and 3-month evaluation period, and magnitude increasing with T stage. They found a high percentage of individuals reporting a loss of control because they could not make themselves understood.

The major complaint of individuals who have been treated for laryngeal cancer is the loss of loudness and the increased effort required to be understood. In addition, when rating their voices, not only the sound of the voice by also the effort required to speak is considered (Woodson et al 1996).

On postsurgical assessment, the quality of voice produced by laryngectomees using tracheo-oesophageal speech has been shown to be much the same as oesophageal speech. Because of longer speaking times, speech is more fluent and intelligible. This fluency has been analysed by having nonprofessional (naive) listeners rate intelligibility and preference. Also voice spectrograms have demonstrated that, although there is no statistically significant difference in fundamental frequency or intensity, the rate of speech production is faster after prosthesis insertion (Heaton et al 1996).

Individuals who have had pharyngeal repair with free jejunum do not achieve consistent voice. Puncture and valve insertion, however, have been shown to allow consistently good, if somewhat gravelly voice. Due to the convolutions, pooling of saliva may be observed above the valve, and this leads to a gurgling quality to the voice on occasions.

Fortunately, there are a variety of devices and procedures that can provide a new source of sound. There are two general categories of sound restoration: mechanical speech aids and alternative 'natural' sound sources. In the former category are the pneumatic and electronic artificial sound sources, and in the latter are oesophageal and tracheo-oesophageal speech (Casper & Colton 1993).

Reconstruction of dentition must be considered for restoration of cosmesis and function following reconstruction of the mandible, with subsequent placement of osseointegrated implants, thereby contributing to articulation; however, there is a debate regarding primary versus secondary placement of osseointegrated implants (McGhee et al 1997).

Sounds affected following glossectomy include vowels requiring a high or frontal tongue position. Additionally, consonants requiring the use of the tongue will be misarticulated.

Defective hearing disrupts human communication, giving rise to anxiety, frustration, stress, isolation, loss of self esteem, even loss of livelihood for the individual with a reduced capacity to receive and interpret sound. Additionally, as we live in families and communities, the effects of hearing loss are not restricted to the impaired individual. Those who associate with that person, especially those who are very close, are affected and prone to many of the same emotions and stresses (Brooks 1989).

REFERENCES

Brooks D N 1989 Adult aural rehabilitation. Chapman & Hall, London
Cahart R 1961 Auditory training. In: Davis H Holt (ed) Hearing and deafness. Rhinehart & Winston, New York
Casper J K, Colton R H 1993 Clinical manual for laryngectomy and head and neck cancer rehabilitation. Singular Publishing Group, California
Clements K S, Rassekh C K, Serkaly H, Hokanson J A, Calhoun K H 1997 Communication

after laryngectomy: an assessment of patient satisfaction. Archives of Otolaryngology – Head and Neck Surgery 123(5): 493–496

Colangelo L A, Logemann J A, Pauloski B R, Pelzer J R, Rademaker A W 1996 T stage and functional outcome in oral and oropharyngeal cancer patients. Head and Neck 18(3): 259–268

Crary M A, Glowasky A L 1996 Using botulinum toxin A to improve speech and swallowing function following total laryngectomy. Archives of Otolaryngology – Head and Neck Surgery 122(7): 760–767

D'Antonio L L, Long S A, Robinson E B, Zimmerman G, Petti G, Chonkich G 1996 Factors related to quality of life and functional status in 50 patients with head and neck cancer. Laryngoscope 106: 1084–1088

Debruyne F, Delaere P, Wouters J, Uwents P 1994 Acoustic analysis of tracheo-oesophageal versus oesophageal speech. The Journal of Laryngology and Otology 108: 325–328

Hawkes M, Keene M, Alberti P W 1990 Clinical otoscopy, 2nd edn. Churchill Livingstone, London

Heaton J M, Parker A J 1994 In vitro comparison of the Gronigen high resistance, Gronigen low resistance and Provox speaking valves. The Journal of Laryngology and Otology 108: 321–324

Heaton J M, Sanderson D, Dunsmore I R, Parker A J 1996 In vivo measurements of indwelling tracheo-oesophageal prosthesis in alaryngeal speech. Clinical Otolaryngology 21: 292–296

Isshiki N, Snidecor J C 1965 Air intake and usage in oesphageal speech. Acta Otolaryngologica 59: 559–574

Izdebski K, Reed C G, Ross J C, Hilsinger R L 1994 Problems with tracheoesophageal fistula voice restoration in totally laryngectomized patients: a review of 95 cases. Archives of Otolaryngology – Head and Neck Surgery 122(8): 858–864

Kornblith A B, Zlotolow I M, Gosen J et al 1996 Quality of life of maxillectomy patients using an obturator prosthesis. Head and Neck Journal for the Sciences and Specialities of the Head & Neck 18(4): 323–334

Kwakman J M, Voorsmit R A, Freihofer H P 1997 Improvement in oral function following tumour surgery by a combination of tongue plasty by the Steinhauser technique and osseointegrated implants. Journal of Craniomaxillofacial Surgery 25(11): 15–18

Leder S B, Erskine C M 1997 Voice restoration after laryngectomy: experience with the Blom-Singer extended wear indwelling tracheo-oesophageal voice prosthesis. Head and Neck 19(6): 487–493

McGhee M A, Stern S J, Callan D, Shewmake K, Smith T 1997 Osseointegrated implants in the head and neck patient. Laryngoscope 106: 1084–1088

McIvor J, Evans P F, Perry A, Cheeseman A D 1990 Radiological assessment of post laryngectomy speech. Clinical Radiology 41: 312–316

Pindzola R H, Cain B H 1988 Acceptability ratings of tracheo oesophageal speech. Laryngoscope 98: 394–397

Schliephake H, Nenkam F W, Schmelzeisen R, Varoga B, Schmeller H 1995 Long term quality of life after ablative intraoral tumour surgery. Journal of Craniomaxillofacial Surgery 120(4): 234–249

Singer M I, Blom E D 1980 An endoscopic technique for restoration of voice after laryngectomy. Annals of Otorhinolaryngology 89: 529–533

Sloane P M, Griffin J M, O'Dwyer T P 1991 Esophageal insufflation and videofluoroscopy for evaluation of esophageal speech in laryngectomy patients: clinical implications. Radiology 181: 433–437

Williams S E, Watson J B 1985 Differences in speaking proficiencies in three laryngectomee groups. Archives of Otolaryngology 111: 216–219

Wilson K J W, Waugh A 1996 Ross and Wilson. Anatomy and physiology, 8th edn. Churchill Livingstone, New York

Woodson G E, Rosen C A, Murry T, Madusa R, Wong F, Hengestey A, Robbins K T 1996 Assessing vocal function after chemoradiation for advanced laryngeal carcinoma. Archives of Otolaryngology – Head and Neck Surgery 122(8): 858–864

# 8

# Psychosocial problems

'As a beauty I'm not a great star.
There are others more handsome, by far
But my face – I don't mind it
For I am behind it,
It's the people in front get the jar'

Anthony Euwer

---

KEY POINTS

- Body image
- The limbic system
- Quality of life studies
- Support groups

---

## INTRODUCTION

Many surgical procedures involving the head and neck are disfiguring and result in some loss of function. It is not surprising, therefore, that much of the nursing literature has focused on the concept of body image, and the need to manage patients from this perspective is obvious.

The idea of body image was initially developed by a neurologist (Head 1920) but was perhaps better expressed by Schilder (1935) as 'the picture of our body which we form in our mind, that is to say the way in which our body appears to ourselves … a tri-dimensional image involving interpersonal, environmental and temporal factors'. There is no doubt that from the earliest times youth, facial beauty and communication skills have played an enormous part in society, and no more so than today when, supported by the mass media and advertising, these qualities are almost worshipped. It is not surprising, therefore, that any alteration to what is perceived as attractive can cause major psychological problems when it happens.

Altered body image can be seen as any significant alteration occurring outside the realms of expected human development. For example, pregnancy and ageing involve physical changes that are acceptable to most people whereas disfigurement due to disease or surgery is not so well toler-ated. Moreover, a change in body image may well affect the way the patient copes with the underlying problem (Bailey & Clarke 1989).

Head and neck patients are at particular risk because so many important functions are related to the area such as sight, sound, smell, taste, eating and communication. The disease process itself may lead to facial palsy, dis-charge and facial disfigurement, and the visibility of prostheses such as tracheostomy tubes, orbital, nasal and auricular prostheses present their own particular anxieties. The effects of radiotherapy may also cause changes in body image: radiation field marks on the skin are visible and cannot be covered with makeup during the treatment, and eating, speaking and swallowing may be difficult. Patients may feel stigmatised and experi-ence a range of psychological and behavioural difficulties.

## ANATOMY AND PHYSIOLOGY

Emotional behaviour and motivational drives are determined by the lim-bic system. This is a functionally related group of structures forming a fringe on the medial side of each hemisphere. These structures are many synapses away from the primary sensory and motor pathways and receive information from the overlying cortex which, after processing, is directed back to the cortex. The limbic system comprises parts of the frontal lobe on either side, namely the cingulate gyrus, the hippocampus, the septum, the amygdaloid nucleus and the anterior thalamic nucleus (Fig. 8.1).

The limbic system is thought to be the site of generation of emotional tone but emotional expression resulting from this is mediated by the hypo-thalamus through the autonomic and somatic systems.

## ASSESSMENT

In common with all surgical specialties, optimal rehabilitation for the head and neck patient begins in the preoperative period and continues postoper-atively. In the pretreatment phase a thorough psychosocial assessment includes a psychiatric history and mental status examination as well as appraisal of marital, family, financial, spiritual and vocational problems. Quality of life (QL) studies can be a useful means of gathering this baseline data and they can be repeated in the evaluation phase. These means of assessment will be discussed later in the chapter but essentially they com-prise a snapshot in time of the patient's perspective of his or her quality of life. A number of investigators have attempted such studies in head and neck cancer patients (Aaronson et al 1993, Cella et al 1993) and it would be reasonable to select the best features of each to form a complete assessment tool.

(a)                                                 (b)

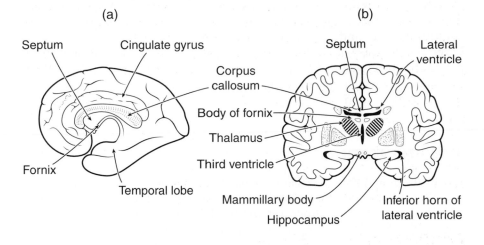

**Figure 8.1**   The limbic system of the brain shown in (a) the medial surface of the right cerebral hemisphere and (b) a frontal section through the juction of the third and lateral ventricles.

## PLANNING

It is clinically evident that many cancer patients develop psychological difficulties. In the case of head and neck patients most problems stem from the fact that the patient's body image is radically altered by the disease itself or the associated treatment. Price (1990) points out that the idea of altered body image is often mentioned in care plans of patients undergoing radical surgery but that nurses may only be able to offer some vague and non-specific form of 'body image care intervention'. Several authors have proposed screening methods (Zabora et al 1990, Anderson 1994) which highlight three areas which need to be considered from a clinical point of view:

- patient variables such as medical and psychiatric comorbidity, social support, socioeconomic status and psychological coping resources (optimism, fighting spirit, hardiness, etc.)
- disease and treatment variables; in general the more treatment modalities are experienced the more likely a patient is to suffer from psychological stress
- communication between the patient and the team.

It is difficult to think of an area of care that would benefit more from a multidisciplinary approach in the planning phase than head and neck cancer care. Edwards et al (1997), however, suggest a depressing picture in this respect. They showed that in the UK, almost a half of consultants had no access to a joint clinic, 40% had no access to a nurse specialist and 35% no contact with counselling services.

It seems almost a matter of common sense to involve specialist nurses, dental hygienists, speech therapists, dieticians, medical social workers, support groups and any other relevant agencies as soon as possible. Indeed, in the case of laryngectomy a presurgical visit by a laryngectomy patient has been reported by patients to be helpful (Casper & Colton 1993). In practice, however, this needs to be very carefully managed, as selection of both patients and visitors is crucial, as of course is the matching of the two!

## IMPLEMENTATION

The traditional nursing models for nursing care based on activities for living offer little scope to develop the need for body image assessment and care (Roper et al 1990). Other nursing models such as Roy's stress adaptation model (Roy 1984) allow more scope and suggest that nursing care can be administered according to how patients adapt to the stressors which affect their internal environment (major surgery) and their external environment (being away from family, losing their job). Clearly the nurse's role is to help patients to adapt to their body image changes, and it goes without saying that this must start by showing the patient unconditional positive regard, which in itself will increase the self-esteem of the patient.

The stress coping model can be used to observe specific behaviours on each postoperative day to indicate how patients are coping. The optimum time for nurses to assist patients in accepting any defects following head and neck surgery are on postoperative days 4–6. By this time the patients have developed affective and physiological coping mechanisms for dealing with stress (Dropkin 1989). These coping strategies are based on the increased use of self-care techniques and social interaction with other patients. Unfortunately, many patients cope well with their altered body image while they have the support of hospital staff, but in the community they may feel isolated and unable to care for their defect, particularly if they need to maintain stomas and feeding regimes. Many patients are reassured by an open-door policy on the ward, and of course close liaison between hospital and community staff is imperative.

The process of acceptance of surgical alteration to body image is characterised by five steps (Bailey & Clarke 1989):

1. accepting the appearance of the site
2. touching and exploring the area
3. learning to care for the defect
4. developing independence and competence to care for the wound site
5. reintegrating the new body image and adjusting to the altered lifestyle.

Practical suggestions pre- and postoperatively such as the use of cosmetic camouflage, a well-fitting prosthesis and suitable clothing, such as filter scarves for laryngectomy patients, are vital to the rehabilitation process. Self-help groups also provide practical help and assist in the socialisation process.

## EVALUATION

The traditional method of reporting the results of treatment for head and neck cancer is to analyse the survival and the rate of side effects from treatment (Gotay & Moore 1992). Patients often have to adapt their lifestyle considerably because of changes in swallowing, speech, breathing or appearance (Langius et al 1994). The impact of such dysfunction on the patients' psychosocial wellbeing or quality of life (QL) can be quite marked but it is not usually investigated or quantified.

The first study to provide a QL index for head and neck cancer was a cross-sectional study (Drettner & Ahlbom 1983). Since then most head and neck QL studies have tended to focus on changes in physical or social functioning, which are components in the multidimensional construct that is quality of life, but do not really reflect the true overall measure that patients identify with.

Dropkin (1989) developed a scale to measure the perception of severity of visible disfigurement and dysfunction after head and neck cancer surgery. She asked 100 registered nurses to rate the disfigurement and dysfunction potential of 11 surgical procedures in terms of body image alteration that patients experience. Interestingly, nurses rated hemilaryngectomy patients as having no body image alteration and total laryngectomy patients as having severe body image alteration.

A practical, working definition of quality of life is the discrepancy between the perceived reality of what one has, and what one wants or expects, or has had (Ochs et al 1988). This is called the gap theory (Ferrans 1990). The greater the gap between one's perceived reality and one's expectations, the greater the dissatisfaction with one's lot.

During the 1990s there was a phenomenal increase in QL-related activity in cancer research. In 1993 alone there were 250 related papers published, 18 of which involved head and neck cancer. Only two of these were prospective in design (Morton 1995). This study shows that life satisfaction improves significantly with time after successful treatment for head and neck cancer. The principal determinants of life satisfaction are pain, dysphagia and difficulty with speech. Patients with a higher life satisfaction at diagnosis tend to be among those with a higher score later. The data apply to survivors. Patients with active recurrent disease were not included. Despite considerable disability within the group, life satisfaction improves as a result of treatment initiatives. The treatment modality did not determine life satisfaction, but specific operations were not examined statistically.

In view of the association of life satisfaction with dysphagia and speech difficulty, it is possible that glossectomy and the use of flaps are important determinants of life satisfaction. Certainly a significant association between type of surgery and performance rating of speech, diet and eating has been demonstrated (List et al 1990). The scale used in this study was easy to administer and included subscales measuring understandability of speech, normalcy of diet and eating in public.

It is the change in physical functioning that the patients notice, and from their point of view it is probably not the operation but the perceived impact on lifestyle that is important. In that event, the measures and general support given to the patient postoperatively in respect of rehabilitation of swallowing and speech becomes critical.

REFERENCES

Aaronson N K, Ahmedzai S, Bergman B et al 1993 The European Organisation for research and Treatment of Cancer QLQ C30: a quality of life instrument for use in international clinical trials in oncology. Journal of the National Cancer Institute 85: 365–376
Anderson B L 1994 Surviving cancer. Cancer 74: 1484–1495
Bailey R, Clarke M 1989 Stress and coping in nursing. Chapman & Hall, London
Casper J K, Colton R H 1993 Clinical manual for laryngectomy and head and neck cancer rehabilitation. Singular Publishing Group, California
Cella D F, Tulsky D S, Gray G et al 1993 The Functional Assessment of Cancer Therapy scale: development and validation of the general measure. Journal of Clinical Oncology 11: 570–579
Drettner B, Ahlbom A 1983 Quality of life and state of health for patients with cancer in the head and neck. Acta Otolaryngologica 96: 307–314
Dropkin M J 1989 Coping with disfigurement and dysfunction after head and neck cancer surgery: a conceptual framework. Seminars in Oncology Nursing 5: 213–219
Edwards D, Johnson N W, Cooper D, Warnakulasuriya K A A S 1997 Management of cancers of the head and neck in the United Kingdom: questionnaire survey of consultants. British Medical Journal 315: 1589
Ferrans C E 1990 Quality of life: conceptual issues. Seminars in Oncology Nursing 6: 248–254
Gotay C C, Moore T D 1992 Assessing quality of life in head and neck cancer. Quality of Life Research 1: 5–17
Head H 1920 Studies in neurology. Oxford University Press, London
Langius A, Bjorvell H, Lind M G 1994 Functional status and coping in patients with oral and pharyngeal cancer. Head and Neck Surgery 16: 559–568
List M A, Ritter-Sterr C, Lansky S B 1990 A performance status scale for head and neck cancer patients. Cancer 66: 564–569
Morton R P 1995 Life satisfaction in patients with head and neck cancer. Clinical Otolaryngology 20: 499–503
Ochs J, Mulhern R, Kun L 1988 Quality of life assessment in cancer patients. American Journal of Clinical Oncology 11: 415–421
Price B 1990 Body image: nursing care and concepts. Prentice Hall, London
Roper N, Logan W W, Tierney A J 1990 The elements of nursing: a model for nursing based on a model for living, 3rd edn. Churchill Livingstone, Edinburgh
Roy C 1984 Introduction to nursing: an adaptation model, 2nd edn. Prentice Hall, London
Schilder P 1935 The image and appearance of the human body: studies in the constructive energies of the psyche. Kegan Paul, London
Zabora J R, Smith-Wilson R, Fetting J H et al 1990 An efficient method for psychosocial screening of cancer patients. Psychosomatics 31: 192–196

# Index

Videofluoroscopy, swallowing, 80
Viral infections, oral ulcers, 56
Visual examination of wound, 63–66
Vocal cords, 115
Vocal rehabilitation, post-laryngectomy, 129–133
Voice prosthesis, 131, 132

## W

Weight, body, 78–79
Wound, 59–72
  assessment, 62–66
  closure, 66
  healing, 59–62

management
  evaluation, 71
  implementation, 66–71
  intraoral, 48, 70–71
  planning, 66

## X

Xerostomia, 50, 54–55
X-rays, plain, upper airway, 22

## Z

Zygomatic branches of facial nerve, 117